Advance praise for *When Your Child Is Gay:*

"Parenting is never easy, but this is especially so when parents have to navigate relatively unchartered waters. When parents learn a child is gay, they immediately wonder how it will affect the child's future and worry, too, about its impact on the lives of other family members. By collecting lessons learned from other parents of gay and lesbian children, and from the gay adults themselves under forty—and adding insightful commentary from an experienced clinician, Jonathan L. Tobkes, M.D., *When Your Child Is Gay* is poised to become an indispensable resource for families. The book offers straightforward, practical advice from people who have been there that will support parents in parenting and understanding their gay adolescent children."

—Irene S. Levine, PhD
Professor of Psychiatry, NYU School of Medicine,
and author of *Best Friends Forever: Surviving a Breakup
with Your Best Friend*

"Navigating the complexities surrounding having a gay child can be daunting for even the greatest parents. Simple questions like *why* and *how* are just the tip of a very large iceberg for many moms and dads. Ms. Davidson uses her trial-by-fire experiences as a straight mom to provide a complete guide that you'll soon discover can make your journey easier. A beautiful relationship with your gay or questioning son or daughter is just a few pages away."

—Bryce Thomason
Founder, EmptyClosets.com

"As the straight mother of a gay son who came out fifteen years ago in the tenth grade, I wish I could have had Ms. Davidson's book to help me understand my feelings at that time. I found the comments at the end of each chapter by Dr. Tobkes particularly helpful for someone like me who is very liberal, yet still needed to process this when it was my own son."

—Cathy Gold, parent of a gay son

"How parents handle a child's 'coming out,' how they deal with their own preconceived expectations of 'who' and 'what' that child should be, and whether they can unwaveringly love, support, protect, and gently guide their child in a society that has yet to accept alternative lifestyles as normal is crucial. If a gay, lesbian, or bisexual teen could hand their parents a comprehensive manual that would help them understand, navigate, and wisely deal with the challenges that both they and their parents face, that guidebook would be *When Your Child Is Gay* by Wesley C. Davidson and Jonathan L. Tobkes, MD, a psychiatrist affiliated with The New York-Presbyterian/Weill Cornell Medical Center in Manhattan—who also happens to be gay. Combining advice from parents and teens who've 'been there' with guidance from a doctor who has not only accepted his sexuality, but celebrates it, *When Your Child Is Gay* will make a bumpy ride a whole lot smoother."

—Phyllis Schneider has served as editor in chief of *YM* magazine and fiction and teen features editor at *Seventeen*, and she was a contributing editor at *Parents* magazine. She is the co-author of *Straight Talk on Women's Health: How to Get the Health Care You Deserve!* and has written extensively about adult and children's health for numerous national magazines.

WHEN YOUR CHILD IS GAY

WHAT YOU NEED TO KNOW

Wesley C. Davidson
and Jonathan L. Tobkes, MD

STERLING
New York

STERLING
New York

An Imprint of Sterling Publishing Co., Inc.
1166 Avenue of the Americas
New York, NY 10036

© 2016 by Wesley C. Davidson and Jonathan L. Tobkes

ISBN 978-1-4549-1936-0

Distributed in Canada by Sterling Publishing Co. Inc.
c/o Canadian Manda Group, 664 Annette Street
Toronto, Ontario, Canada M6S 2C8
Distributed in the United Kingdom by GMC Distribution Services
Castle Place, 166 High Street, Lewes, East Sussex, England BN7 1XU

33614057583121

For information about custom editions, special sales, and premium
and corporate purchases, please contact Sterling Special Sales at
800-805-5489 or specialsales@sterlingpublishing.com.

Manufactured in Canada

2 4 6 8 10 9 7 5 3 1

www.sterlingpublishing.com

To our son, whose story became ours.

—WESLEY

To my parents, Susan and Jeffrey Tobkes, who have done
so much more for me than "just getting their lines right."
I am forever grateful to be their son.

—JONATHAN

Contents

Foreword

WHEN WESLEY DAVIDSON asked me to write the foreword to the book she had coauthored with Jonathan Tobkes, M.D., I was honored and thrilled: The personal experience, perceptive insight, and extensive research that she and Jonathan have poured into this book make it both an incredibly compelling and helpful read for parents—or anyone out there—who would like to learn more about the dual processes of raising a gay or lesbian child and growing up as gay or lesbian.

As many of you know, the unfortunate reality is that growing up lesbian, gay, bisexual, or transgender (LGBT) can be, and is often, very tough. Many LGBT youth experience rejection by members of their families and communities. I can testify to this fact, both in my own personal experiences growing up as a young gay and also in the multitude of stories that other gay and lesbian young people have shared with me over the years. In many ways, however, acceptance is also a common theme that unites the narratives of multitudes of well-adjusted gay and lesbian youth everywhere. By reading Wesley and

Jonathan's book, you are taking the first step toward becoming a more educated and accepting parent, friend, teacher, or mentor to the LGBT people in your life.

When I, myself, came out in my early teens, I experienced both sides of the coin: acceptance and rejection. I was blessed to have parents who loved me for me and accepted me. To this day, I am deeply grateful to them for being so unwaveringly supportive from day 1—I truly don't think I would be the person I am now if not for their response. However, my grandparents had a very different response. Deeply Catholic, my sexuality was at odds with their faith, and though they loved me deeply, they struggled with my sexuality and preferred that it stay closeted. Additionally, not everyone in my community was as accepting as my parents. I faced name-calling at school, and many times I felt ashamed of myself because of my sexuality. These challenges, though extremely painful at times, ultimately became a major force in shaping my personality and my worldview. Over time, my grandparents' views evolved, and they came to accept my sexuality. This culminated in one of the most emotional moments in my quest to support The Trevor Project by becoming the first openly LGBT person to climb the "Seven Summits." Before I set off to climb Everest, my grandmother called me and told me she was proud of my project and asked how she could donate to support The Trevor Project, an organization that provides life-saving services to tens of thousands of LGBTQ (the Q is alternatively interpreted as queer or questioning) youth every year. Had my grandparents had access to a book such as Wesley and

Jonathan's when I came out, their journey to acceptance and support might have been much shorter.

Everyone faces challenges in life, but for gay and lesbian young people, ordinary and simple tasks like changing in the locker room or putting on your outfit for school can result in name-calling, bullying, harassment, and worse. The worst of my experiences paled in comparison to what many young gay and lesbian youth go through on a daily basis around the country. The statistics are chilling: 90 percent of LGBT students hear anti-LGBT comments in school, and one in four LGBT students has been physically attacked by another student due to their sexual orientation. What is even more terrifying is that roughly 34 percent of LGBT youth report that they experienced physical violence from their parents because of their sexuality, and 26 percent of LGBT youth were forced to leave their home because of it.

But there is a bright side: LGBT youth with highly supportive families and communities are significantly more likely to have higher self-esteem and acknowledge having suicidal thoughts at dramatically lower rates. Through books such as this one, which teach people how to be more supportive, we can change the world for LGBT youth. Our society would be a healthier, more supportive one for all were this book required reading for everyone. At a minimum, it should be required reading for anyone who is LGBT or has an LGBT person in their lives. Wesley and Jonathan's instructive chapters provide a brilliant guide through what can be a very difficult and confusing process for both an LGBT youth and those who care about that person. Looking back, my own experience growing up LGBT would have been less painful had I been able to read this book earlier in my life, and I certainly wish that members of my community and family had had access to such a book. *When Your Child Is Gay: What You Need to Know* will change your life, but more importantly, it will help you change the lives of the LGBT people you know and love.

—*Cason Crane*

Founder of The Rainbow Summits Project

LogoTV's Youth Trailblazer Honoree, 2013
Princeton University 2017

Preface: The Find

I n late October 1996, while picking up our son James's room, I moved a composition book from which fell a folded sheet of notebook paper. I didn't mean to look at it, but I did. It was a love note, my son's name entwined with another boy's, surrounded with a heart. Hadn't I just driven him across town for the umpteenth time to see a female classmate whom he said he was going to marry? I was stunned, to say the least.

Covering my tracks, I folded the piece of paper along its original creases and slipped it back into the comp book. I hoped he wouldn't notice that it had been moved. It wasn't my custom to invade my son's space, and my son knew that and trusted me because of it. I didn't want that to change. Yet, despite my best intentions, I now felt irresistibly compelled to snoop. I just couldn't help myself. I slid off his bed and looked under it. All I found were summer camp letters and birthday cards stacked in size 10M shoe boxes; a gnawed dog bone from Daisy, our German short-haired pointer; a pencil that needed sharpening; and more dust bunnies than I cared to count. I lifted up his mattress and felt along where the bed met the wall. I came up dry again.

Now I was on a mission. I wanted to find some evidence of the part of my son that he had kept hidden from me. Or that perhaps I had kept hidden from myself. I flung open the doors to his closet and looked for I'm not sure what. I noticed that, for a teenage boy, his closet looked as if it were ready for military inspection, and everything was color-coordinated. Did this mean something? I could detect the fragrance of his familiar Ralph Lauren cologne, and yet, at the bottom, his frequently sweated-up tennis shoes made it smell like a gym locker, which was all straight boy.

Well, was he gay or wasn't he?

As I left, I passed the doors at the bottom of his stairs: One led to the yard and the other to the garage. Either one could usher clandestine suitors into his bedroom. I imagined these doors as secret passageways perfectly designed to accommodate unseen late night rendezvous. Our bedroom was on the opposite side of the house so his companions would pass unnoticed.

My feelings of confusion and powerlessness made me feel as if I were having an out-of-body experience. The slow, uncertain walk down the stairs felt like sloshing through floodwaters.

Spent and anxious, I calmed my nerves with a ritual cup of afternoon tea. I opened a red plaid box of shortbread cookies, and ate not one, not two, but five in a row, and like Proust, I let the cookies unlock thoughts of times long past.

I was introduced to shortbread by my maternal grandmother, who was thought to be a lesbian, although no one
seemed to know for sure. I found this out after she died in
1966. She was divorced and always lived with single women;
one friend—probably partner—had a beautiful fieldstone farm
we would visit in Bucks County. It never occurred to me that
these ladies could be lesbians; it didn't matter to me. I was
loved by all.

My grandmother was respected by everyone and raised me
while my mother worked. She supported herself and had been
an executive at Elizabeth Arden as well as a model for artist
Howard Chandler Christy, whose murals grace the famous
New York restaurant Café des Artistes. She ran a girls' camp in
Sutton, New Hampshire, primarily for society girls from Philadelphia's Main Line region, because "rich girls don't know
how to play." Gloria Steinem could have learned a lot from her!

Nanny's recipe for "slightly burnt eggs," printed in her local
newspaper, is also preserved in its original writing, now quite
yellowed, in my scrapbook. The scrapbook also has her star-
tling tip that spit works just as well as mascara! She allowed my
mother, a good student, to be excused from school on Wednes-
days, when there was no after-school sports, to attend the theater. What's not to like?

I wondered if Nanny had a tough time going against society's norms. Would my son have a tough time being gay? And
who should know about this? Should I risk telling my conservative southerners-in-law who are customarily supportive of
my children, only to then watch them recoil in horror when

they hear the news that James is gay? If I share my suspicions with a close friend, will she, with one-too-many cocktails, inadvertently gossip?

Should I say anything to my husband? How would John take this news? I didn't want to burden him with my worries that would become his worries. He takes a 5:15 a.m. train to work. He can't afford to lose sleep. What about my eight-year-old daughter Ann? Isn't she too young to understand?

In my mind, my son James left that morning at a quarter to eight as a heterosexual. What would he be to me when he walked back in? What would I say to him, especially since I gained information from snooping? How would I act? Would I feel the same way about him? And maybe it wasn't true. Maybe someone put that in his book without him knowing. Maybe that person thought my son was gay even though he wasn't. Maybe this was just a phase he was going through. Maybe I'd better not mention my hunches to James or anyone else in case this is all just a big mistake. Oh please, God, please let this be a mistake!

These were the thoughts, fears, and questions that churned through my mind that very first day. Seventeen years later, my son and I have arrived at a new and more accepting place. We are both out of denial. We don't have everything resolved, but we can talk to each other when we're having issues. With help from PFLAG, a therapist, and unconditional love, we have talked our way through issues that I never dreamed I could have approached the day I was rifling through James's room in that so-long-ago, and oh-so-revealing, October.

I'm not shocked anymore. I feel comfortable about James's gay friends. I've been to gay bars with James. Our family has entertained his boyfriends in our homes and reveled in the fact that James has had his arms around a lover on our den sofa. I have also cried when a lover has jilted him.

And while I have come a long way from that place in the years since discovering my son was gay, it hasn't been easy. Had there been a way for me to speak to myself now, back then, if there had been others, who had been down this road before, to inform my journey, how much easier it would have been, for me and for my son. Looking back, it would have been so much easier if I had known others who had gay sons and could have guided me. That is why I am writing this book for parents of all gender-fluid children, be they gay, lesbian, bisexual, pansexual, or transgender.

My journey has led me to a better understanding of my situation, and sharing with others who have been there and done that has enhanced that understanding enormously. So I decided to open up a dialogue with parents and kids across the country, in the hopes that the understanding that they've gained through their journey might help others to cover the territory more easily.

I certainly had no role models and neither do most parents, so they shouldn't expect themselves to be immediately equipped to handle the additional responsibilities of parenting gay kids while they are trying to take care of themselves. Because it's so important for parents to know what to say to their gay and lesbian children, my coauthor Jonathan Tobkes, MD, who happens to be gay and is legally married in New York State, will, in each issue-oriented chapter, take the parents' emotional pulse and comment on the feelings, normalizing their behavior. Dr. Tobkes, a cum laude Yale graduate who teaches and supervises psychiatry residents at the New York-Presbyterian/Weill Cornell Medical Center, offers suggestions for parents and their children to resolve conflict so they gain better understanding and improve their relationship. His tips are based on his work with clients: gay, lesbian, bisexual, and straight.

Parenting a child is hard enough. Compound that with worrying about your child being bullied, either online or in school, being legally fired in a job owing to his sexual orientation, and not being accepted by a society where homophobia is alive and well. In spite of the significant strides made on the civil rights front, there is still hatred.

You will find in this book parents who never thought they would be able to understand their gay child and know what it feels like to be gay. But with love, time, and patience, they were able to overcome their doubts. Whether they live in the Bible Belt, the Northeast, or the liberal West, they share their stories so you may learn what worked, or didn't work, in raising a healthy and happy gay/lesbian child. Not only will you find yourself more confident and happier, but it will spill over to your child.

This book does not claim to be a *one-size-fits-all* approach—the script varies, but parents, gays, and lesbians will profit from those who seem to be dealing with similar issues. You will find takeaway messages in each chapter in a section called "The Doctor Is In," as well as common threads throughout so you won't feel as if you're floundering on your own.

Your child needs understanding, unconditional love, and empathy. You may need to adjust your expectations as I did for my child. Together, with the aid of those in the know, you can be a more effective parent right now and in the future. It may take a village to raise a child, but it always starts with a caring parent.

—*Wesley C. Davidson*

WHEN
YOUR CHILD
IS GAY

· 1 ·

DENIAL TO DISCOVERY

"To regret one's own experiences is to arrest one's own development. To deny one's own experience is to put a lie into the lips of one's own life. It is no less than a denial of the soul."

—Irish author Oscar Wilde (1854–1900)

E VEN CARING AND open-minded parents can find themselves at odds with their child's coming out. The child you
thought you knew now has (and may have always had) a
new sexual identity. This earth-shaking news can produce in
parents several uncomfortable feelings such as shame, fear,
guilt, and loss, which bleed like a Rorschach test into other
areas of life. Denial is the most common initial emotion that
the parents I spoke with experienced.

If denial were what I was initially feeling, with its tentacles
of overwhelming issues, it was nowhere as strong as what my
son was feeling. The collateral damage of denial can be so
overwhelming that it mirrors the symptoms of clinical post-
traumatic stress disorder (PTSD). Not relegated to soldiers,
PTSD is an equal opportunity destroyer: *Fear, shock, helpless-
ness, stress,* and *extreme sadness*—these are all words that parents
and their gay children use to describe their experiences in the
denial zone.

Looking back at the days following my *big snoop,* I must
have been in denial. Our son continued to see "his girlfriend"

across town. As long as he hung out with her, I felt somewhat confident that he was an average teen with active hormones attracting him to the opposite sex. If this situation were to take place nowadays, I might consider the possibility that he was questioning his sexual orientation or that he could be bisexual.

I never questioned him about the heart I found on the sly. How would I have brought it up? I would have been embarrassed to initiate a conversation. This was not your usual "birds and bees" talk—it was inferring that my child was gay. Talk about opening up Pandora's Box! I had a close, loving, and trusting relationship with my son, and I wanted to keep it that way. So I muzzled myself.

Somewhere in the recesses of my mind, however, I must have known without knowing, in that way that you do, that my son was gay, because I mentioned it to a therapist. The therapist reassured me that my fears were probably unfounded.

"Wesley, give your son the benefit of the doubt," he said casually. "He's probably got a crush on an older guy, which is not uncommon." Now, I know, of course, that same-sex experimentation is normal and does not mean you're gay. I immediately thought, of course, I'm being silly. After all, if an authority figure says it isn't so, then my hunch must be wrong. And so I returned to my blissful state of denial, as many parents do. But I have learned that knowing is always better than not knowing, and when it comes to parenting a gay teen, you have to trust your instincts and address the situation so that you can truly know your child and offer him or her the needed support.

The interviewees below have all successfully come to terms with their initial denial.

Pamela, Mother, Sixty-Five

"I was devastated, completely shocked, and in denial," said Pamela Testone, mother of Glennda Testone, Executive Director of the LGBT Center in Manhattan.

Pamela's first reaction to Glennda's coming out was complete denial. How could she be gay—she dates boys! Glennda had always been a "girly-girl." She was captain of the cheerleading team at school and dated the captain of the basketball team. Then she lived in New Jersey with a boyfriend for *four* years.

Glennda, now thirty-nine, did well in school, majoring in Women's Studies at Ohio State. When she graduated, she became Media Director at GLAAD (Gay & Lesbian Alliance Against Defamation), an organization that fights discrimination against the gay, lesbian, bisexual, transgender population in the media. She is currently the Executive Director of the second largest LGBT Center in the United States in New York City's Chelsea neighborhood. Glennda was twenty-seven when she came out to her mother, which may have made the news a bit harder to digest. Pamela had just that much more time to think of her daughter as a heterosexual.

Glennda's news whipped up a familiar tempest of anxiety for her mother. It was verbal cyanide to Pamela, causing seismic changes in her family. The Testones' well-ordered life was suddenly thrown off-kilter, and Glennda's and Pamela's formerly loving relationship changed, at least initially. Mother and daughter had been close. Now, with withered hopes for Glennda's mainstream future that Pamela thought would include a husband and children, she felt as if a wedge had come between them. They fought all the time and were seemingly constantly angry at each other. Figuratively, it was a slugfest.

Pamela worried that her relationship with Glennda would never be close again and that ultimately they would be alienated from each other. When Glennda brought home partners, not once, but twice, this added to the tension in the Testones' house. The visits with partners seemed to just underscore the fact that Glennda was actually a lesbian, and Pamela felt that Glennda was thrusting her lifestyle in her face, which was tough for Pamela to accept. Although Pamela's career was that of a social worker for gay-friendly organizations and her husband, a retired school superintendent, had a gay nephew they both liked, she was still daunted by her daughter's changed future, one that she had never wanted or imagined for her.

Although overcoming denial is not easy and has no predictable time frame, Pamela estimates that it took from one to two years to get over her denial. In retrospect, she realizes now that she was more worried about her relationship with Glennda than she was about Glennda being a lesbian—there was a threat to the mother's and daughter's close relationship, which was previously close.

"There was upheaval," confessed Pamela, "but Vito [her

husband] and I stuck it out, and we would visit with Glennda
five or six times a year. You have to get right with yourself.
What I learned is that if you love your child, all will be okay in
the end." By confiding to close friends she could trust, Pamela
found positivity. Journaling helped her see behavior patterns
that she needed to change; it was a good method of venting as
well as a way to record progress toward a better relationship
with Glennda.

"I read books about relationships with adult children, such
as Deborah Tannen's *I Only Say This Because I Love You* [Random
House, 2002] as well as *Walking on Eggshells: Navigating the
Delicate Relationship Between Adult Children and Their Parents*
[Random House, 2008]. They helped. What you have to realize
is, it's not about you."

When I last saw Pamela Testone, she was on a viral video
speaking about her journey to acceptance, on the very night
that Glennda received an award from the LGBT Center where
she has been the Executive Director since 2009. Both of them
were beaming.

My Experience with Denial

Learning that your child is gay is a lightning first-jolt to any
parent. You don't expect the news; parents don't anticipate that
their "baby" could be gay. I can't say that I was as broadsided as
Pamela, because I wasn't *told* by my son that he was gay. I had
gotten my first inkling on my own. In my estimation at the

time, our son wasn't old enough to know about his sexual orientation, whereas Pamela's daughter, in her twenties, was certain. *Golly gee*, I thought at the time, *our son is probably still a virgin*. There were no words to sting, no proclamation of, "Mom, Dad, I'm gay!" There was only a piece of paper to go on, with no other clues in his room. And that meant I could stay in denial as long as I wanted, and so could my son.

Talking about my grandmother in a positive way to James, and including her sexual orientation, never inched him closer to the epiphany I was waiting for. He became depressed, and we suspected he had mononucleosis, but he tested negative.

James never liked school, even nursery school, but at least he *attended*. In tenth grade, he stopped going to high school. His psychologist (and later on, James himself) told me that he was teased by his classmates. Interestingly enough, my son told me why they were teasing him; they called him "gay." Yet he would not admit he was gay to me. The silence and my denial were literally making him sick.

His depression became my sadness. It is horrible to watch your child sink into lethargy, watching *The Price Is Right* in his pajamas when he should be in school. Or spending many hours in his room swaddled in blankets, eventually dropping out of school altogether.

Continuing to hang out with girls, and in a romance with a girl in the eleventh grade, James took another full year to come out. I don't think that my denial and my obvious desire to reject the truth about my son helped him to stand on his truth. I don't think it was coincidental that it happened after he split for North Carolina first, and then to California, where he had boyfriends. I didn't have to ask him at that point if he was gay.

In the past, whenever I asked, he didn't like being singled out, defied self-affirmation, and would explode at the question. I never pressed the issue, but today, seeing him in the sun of self acceptance, and out of denial myself, I realize that acknowledging reality is better than avoiding the truth.

Eileen, Mother, Fifty-Two

"In hindsight, the whole subject of whether Sean was gay or not probably was complete denial all along. Why could I not see what others clearly saw in him? Is that denial? Maybe, or is it just a mother's love and instinct to protect her child?"

Eileen Kelly believed that unless her son told her flat out that he was gay, then he was straight. This classic denial response bought her time.

Growing up, Eileen, now fifty-two, never heard the word "gay."

"I went to Catholic school taught by nuns," she explains with a touch of embarrassment now. "The school, church, and the village were all within a one-mile radius of my home. I thought everyone was white, Irish, and Catholic, and that we'd all grow up and have large families just like the families we came from in Boston. I didn't know that other families had divorce, alcoholism, and other afflictions. It wasn't discussed."

Neither, apparently, was her sister's lesbianism. Eileen's mother suspected that Eileen's sister was a lesbian and would ask Eileen and her younger sister to spy on their closeted lesbian sister and her partner and report back. Bob, their father, was never told, because Eileen was convinced that the truth would not only hurt, but kill him.

"My two 'macho' brothers and I finally figured it out, and I was the one that was selected to talk to my lesbian sister and tell her that we knew and that we very much wanted her to be open and that there was nothing we would not do for her and her partner." Eileen's three children knew their aunty was gay and loved her just the same.

"I felt badly that I had been so blind and didn't recognize she was a lesbian until after she was forty," Eileen told me with a tinge of regret in her voice. Eileen's sister finally came out—about three or four years prior to Eileen's son. And when he did, she thought long and hard about her sister.

"Knowing how my sister was closeted all those years, it didn't sit well with me, and I certainly did not want the same thing for my son," said Eileen. And it was this experience that helped Eileen to begin to make her way out of the land of denial.

They tried to coax Sean to come out, but Sean wasn't ready. On the following Thanksgiving, however, Sean dropped the bomb when the family was visiting Grandpa on Cape Cod. Only his sister Kathy knew that Sean was gay because he had confided in her three weeks before coming out to his mother.

Sean, Kathy, Maureen, and Eileen were all playing darts together. Dad was watching television in a separate room.

"Don't you have something to say?" his sister had urged him, wanting Sean to tell Eileen the truth about himself. And then Sean told his mother that he was gay.

"My first reaction was panic," said Eileen. "My throat went dry, my mind went numb. I had to take a few moments to compose myself." This is a common visceral reaction. Even though Eileen had wanted her son to come out, when he finally did, she was flooded by doubts for herself and her child and responded with a whole new kind of denial.

"I must have spent two months becoming completely numb," Eileen explained. "I was angry. What would being gay mean to his life? Would he have to lead a dual life like my sister? As Sean didn't find the nerve to tell his dad until three months later, I bore the burden." It took Sean about three months to tell his father, but when he did, his dad readily accepted him, contrary to what he thought would happen.

Eventually, Sean became more comfortable with his gayness. At the end of his junior year in high school, Sean went to a private performing arts high school. The transition was easy: He lived in a dorm with thirty-five young men, only two of whom were straight. Now Sean is at the New England Conservatory, after attending the Manhattan School of Music for four years. As there is a large population of gays who are accepted in the arts, Eileen doesn't worry as much about Sean being harassed. Eileen herself found solace in PFLAG and is now the Co-Chair of the Greater PFLAG in Boston. She, having been granted permission by Sean and the rest of the family, is out about her son's sexual orientation. The family has left denial behind and are moving forward together in the realm of new discovery and truth.

As Eileen and I will attest, keeping sexual orientation under wraps drives a wedge between parent and child, as well as other members of the family. Sean's sister knew he was gay before the rest of the family, just as I sensed that our son was gay before his sister knew. Maintaining a secret as weighty as this one, always trying to hide it from other family members as well as outsiders, is exhausting; whom and what have I told becomes a daily exercise difficult to remember with all its fabrications. It's also untruthful and evasive.

Eileen was used as the stool pigeon in her family to spy on her sister, who was lesbian. If the sister had been able to come out while living under the same roof as her parents, Eileen wouldn't have felt guilty all these years about her sister being closeted, just as my son stayed closeted and couldn't come out until he had left home. Wouldn't it have been better if the dialogue were more open so mother and son could have spoken about their concerns, and I, as a parent, like Eileen, would not have forced myself into believing that as long as my son dated girls, his future would be as I planned?

Sean is fortunate to have accepting parents. Too many lesbian and gay children are rejected by their parents. One such child is Sheila Longren.

Sheila Longren, Daughter, Fifty-Four

"I tried to be straight for eight years—obviously it didn't work."

Sheila Longren is a successful entrepreneur who grew up in a Westchester County bedroom community north of New York City. After Sheila attended camp one summer, her friends began noticing that something about her was different, and they started teasing her about being a lesbian.

When Sheila was sixteen, she kept a bulletin board in her room, as most teens do. But on Sheila's board, there was a calendar called *Firehouse Gay Women* with events and buttons associated with the lesbian community. After finding the bulletin board, her mother, incensed, stabbed the photos with a knife and put the board on Sheila's bed. Her father, "the bleeding heart liberal," was more supportive, but he lived elsewhere, as her parents were divorced.

Trying to fix what she perceived as a "problem," Sheila's mother sent her daughter to a therapist. The therapist said to the mother that Sheila's interest in females was "just a phase" she was experiencing—exactly what her mother wanted to hear. But although Sheila tried to deny it, and never told her mother, she could not shake the feelings she had for other women. And this caused her to feel perpetual disapproval by her mother, because Sheila knew deep down that she would never be whom her mother wanted her to be.

Although Sheila graduated first in her class from State University of New York at Purchase, she was hard pressed to make her mother proud. She spent three years not talking to her mother, as the "L" word was not part of her mother's vocabulary. Even though Sheila was living with her lifetime partner, Karen Saunders, her mother would call and say, "Can we talk, or is *that person* there?"

"That person" still lives with Sheila in an artsy community on the Hudson River. They invest in real estate and are interested in preserving old buildings.

For whatever reasons—her mother's hostility, others' acceptance, societal prejudice against gays—Sheila wanted to be straight but was conflicted. This was particularly evident in 1977, when she was dating a successful bond trader in the Hamptons, where she had a house share. She went out with Jerry for three years, but found herself still irresistibly drawn to women.

Sheila became a classic overachiever, excelling in the testosterone-fueled world of Wall Street, all the while frantically trying to deny her truth, dating men in public and women in secret, all in an attempt to make her mother happy. In 1991, while a Managing Director for Bear Stearns, she finally left the land of denial behind her and decided she could no longer hide.

These days, Sheila doesn't have to deny anything. She's "out there" as president of a financial firm that specializes in counseling same-sex couples who have unique issues such as additional taxation and other unfair lack of benefits. After twenty years on Wall Street, she, a Managing Partner and Chief Financial Partner, says, "I like working with individuals.

It's more rewarding than working with portfolio managers on the institutional side of Wall Street."

Sheila also helps the LGBTQ community through the Point Foundation. It empowers promising top-notch students who are LGBTQ with full scholarships to achieve their full academic and leadership potential. To qualify, scholars are chosen for their demonstrated involvement in the LGBTQ community. The Point Foundation is the most substantive academic award of its kind. Its recipients are matched with mentors from the professional world in fields that are appealing to them.

Like many LGBTQ children who may still feel unsupported by parents, Sheila has found "family" through her work, her lifetime partner, and her identification with the community. However, when I asked Sheila about her mother, she rolled her eyes.

As you can see, parents who are in denial force their kids, such as Sheila, to live in denial as well. This has caused Sheila to look for validation elsewhere: work, community, and a home where she is accepted for herself. Sheila's unmet needs within her original family are now met with her new family.

Our denial, and our child's response to it, and the child's desire to embody the very wishes of their parents, can shape a person's life long-term, as it did with Sheila. Sometimes, gay children are frightened of rejection by their parents once they are found out. Sheila, as we've read, had reason to be scared of her mother's reaction. However, sometimes, as in the following example, parents' unconditional love for their gay child will trump any rejecting behaviors such as scorn or anger.

Who would have thought that Tyler Harvey, raised Pentecostal in the Bible Belt, would have parents who would respond with tolerance?

Tyler Harvey, Son, Seventeen

"I am gay, but my sexuality does not define me. I believe I have a calling from God to help shatter the traditional belief that homosexuality is a sin." Tyler Harvey lives in the Bible Belt of Arkansas. He was raised in the Pentecostal Church where he was taught, at his mother's knee, that homosexuality is a sin. At age seventeen, he came out to a friend. His mother and father found out Tyler was gay through an e-mail message meant for Tyler, about a Gay Pride event. A well-behaved young man, Tyler did not deny it, although he knew he was disappointing his parents' American dream for him: marriage, children, and house with the white picket fence.

To help educate his mother, Tyler gave her the books *Torn: Rescuing the Gospel from the Gays-vs.-Christians Debate* by Justin Lee (Jericho Books, 2012) and *Prayers for Bobby: A Mother's Coming to Terms with the Suicide of Her Gay Son* by Leroy F. Aarons (HarperCollins, 1995). He also suggested that she contact PFLAG, but there was no meeting place near their home in Ft. Smith, Arkansas.

"My mother asked me how long I had known. I think I've known since I was twelve. I just have never been attracted to girls. She also asked me if I was sure. Maybe she didn't want it to be so!"

Yet despite his mother's questions, Tyler found his mother, a maker of fish lures, and his father, who debones chicken at the local Perdue plant, to be accepting. He wishes in a way that he had told them sooner. They "love the sinner, but not the sin," so to speak. Many parents, because of their unconditional love for their child, will find acceptance. "You need to figure out if your family is going to support you; if they're going to be violent and hostile, then don't tell them," cautions Tyler.

"I always acted straight," confessed Tyler, whose younger sister was "just okay" with his coming out. He played clarinet in high school and was good at computers and technology. Now in community college, he lives with his grandmother to be closer to college and church on Sundays. He is not out to his church, as he knows it would be frowned upon, to put it mildly.

Tyler described his former spiritual life as "drowning in my own self-pity," struggling with the lack of understanding in the people around him. Trying to rectify the conflict, he sought out a pastor in a neighboring Pentecostal church. That pastor suggested he "pray away the gay" by attending a conversion camp intended to change the sexual orientation of gays. Tyler had enough sense not to try one.

Organized religion is usually a hiccup to advancing gay

rights and endorsing diversity. It prevents parents from seeing that God loves everyone, including their gay son or daughter, and doesn't regard that child as sinful. For parents who wish to reconcile their faith with their child's sexual orientation, there are organizations found in the Resources section (see page 203) for various religions.

I was never taught that homosexuality was wrong, only that it was caused by a domineering mother and ineffectual father, a mindset of the 1960s. What parent wants to think of himself in this way? So in fact, denial may be easier to cope with. Of course, I now know better, as do psychiatrists and psychologists, who declassified homosexuality as a mental disorder in the 1970s.

Religion, moral codes, and preconceived expectations can all cause parents to deny their child's same-sex orientation and fully accept the child's identity. In "The Doctor Is In" section at the end of the chapter, my coauthor, Jonathan L. Tobkes, M.D., psychiatrist, illustrates why parents deny and gives suggestions for parents to resolve this conflict.

Ashlee Cain, Daughter, Twenty-Two

"Just looking." That's what Ashlee told herself from middle school through college when she ogled good-looking girls. After all, it was the boys who, in her words, "gave her butterflies" and whom she dated. At first, Ashlee rationalized that what attracted her must be the outfit the girl was wearing or the hairdo that she coveted. But it wasn't. It was the whole package, but she had to grow out of her shame and denial to figure out that she was bisexual. Although currently dating the same guy for four years, she still finds herself attracted to women.

Ashlee's mother, Felicia, gave birth to her daughter when she was just fifteen years old. By exercising extraordinarily strict rules, Felicia hoped to make sure that her daughter wouldn't repeat her mistakes. Ashlee, who lives with her mother, brother, and sister in New Jersey, has had to be accountable her whole life: she was expected to do plenty of chores, was grounded when she misbehaved, couldn't date before age sixteen, had to do well in school, and attend the Baptist church.

However, Ashlee didn't find much spirituality in the Baptist religion. "Christianity instilled a lot of guilt, judgment, and fear in me for years," she said. "I've been a much happier person without it." Her mother, now thirty-seven, has also stopped going to church because she didn't agree with judgmental and exclusionary practices not only in her church, but in others as well.

By the time Ashlee entered college, she couldn't brush off her feelings about women. She better understood her attraction but thinks she also harbored shame at this time, so she downplayed her interest in women.

In college, she attended an LGBT support group and

learned a name for what she felt: bisexual. She also was told that you don't have to actually have same-sex relationships to be considered bisexual. Even though there were lesbians in her college as well as "bis," Ashley didn't want her initiation into sleeping with women to be the result of too much alcohol or a hookup (common on her campus), so she bypassed the opportunity time and time again.

Ashlee, an assistant at a midsize publishing company in Manhattan, thinks bisexuals have been given a bum rap by society. They are often considered "half-queer." Lesbians don't care for them because they are "sleeping with the enemy." Straight people think bisexuals are greedy, having voracious appetites for sex with both genders. Others want them to "get off the fence and choose." Are they straight or gay? Straight parents pray that their bisexual son or daughter will choose just one sexual identity, and often they hope for the heterosexual one.

Despite her confirmation as a bisexual, Ashlee has not changed her sexual preference on Facebook since 2009, continuing to identify on the site as heterosexual. This is not typical of the trend of people using Facebook as a platform for coming out.

When she was a sophomore in college, Ashlee told her mother that she was sexually interested in women. Her mother was "cool" with it, as is her boyfriend, whom she met during her freshman year. Ashlee surmises that her mother already knew about her same-sex attraction. This past November,

Ashlee came out to her mother, who simply replied, "I thought we already covered this."

Ashlee is no longer in denial. She knows that she's bisexual and is not afraid to tell others. "As I look at it, it doesn't change who you are," she says. "I'm still moral, kind, responsible. All it changes is your sex life."

Liz R., Daughter, Thirty-One

"It was a gradual process coming out as a lesbian," commented Liz, who until last year, identified as bisexual. During college in Massachusetts and high school in Florida, Liz dated boys, but always, like Ashlee, she felt a pull toward women. When Liz broke up with her boyfriend during her senior year in college, she wondered if she was bisexual. She kept this epiphany to herself except that she "tested the waters" by telling her best friend in high school. (Often, I hear from LGBT people that it is common practice to come out to nonjudgmental friends before coming out to their parents.)

After college graduation, Liz took a job at a daily newspaper in a rural conservative town not far from Scranton, Pennsylvania, for a year. It was during this time that she began her first lesbian relationship. She next moved to New York City, where she has been an editor for three years at a website for TV listings, videos, and entertainment news.

"At first, I gave myself permission to go to lesbian bars, but just on the weekend. Then, it became more often. I didn't tell anyone." In fact, her office friends, who wanted to fix her up on a date with a man, didn't know she was gay until Liz mentioned that she had a girlfriend.

Liz's parents didn't know until 2012 that Liz was a lesbian. There was no formal coming out. Her mother accidentally discovered Liz's secret as she was looking for photos on Liz's digital camera. She found pictures of other lesbians, and events for the Human Rights Campaign, America's largest civil rights organization that works for LGBT equality. Horrified, she asked Liz, "Who are *these* people?" Her mother next asked her daughter if she was bisexual. Liz, knowing full well she was a lesbian but not wanting to disappoint her mother, answered affirmatively. Her mother also inquired, hoping that her dreams for her daughter wouldn't be dashed, if she planned to date men.

During that year, Liz was in two lesbian relationships, each one lasting about six months. For the next two years, Liz told her mother, sixty-six, and her father, sixty-eight, that she was bisexual to make it easier on herself, but she knew better.

Acceptance during the years of 2012–2014 was not in Liz's parents' vocabulary, nor was the "L word." Liz let them think she was bisexual until she came out after 2014 as a lesbian. "I didn't speak to my parents for a week," she said. Then the e-mails from them would start. "They'd be calm for a while, and then, all of a sudden, there'd be a flurry of derogatory calls and e-mails aimed at my status. Ad nauseum, they would make comments such as 'you haven't met the right boy yet' (denial), 'you're destroying the family,' 'what will our friends think?', 'don't tell the relatives, particularly the ninety-year-old British aunt!' (shame), 'we never should have sent you to such a gay-friendly college,' and 'your mother isn't sleeping' (guilt).

Interestingly enough, Liz had run the gamut of these issues and others, such as fear, loss, and anger. To try to gain acceptance from her parents, Liz ordered books that she thought would contribute to an understanding of what it means to be gay. There were classics such as *Beyond Acceptance: Parents of Lesbian and Gays Talk About Their Experiences* by Griffin, W. Wirth, and A. Wirth (St. Martin's Griffin, 1997) and *Straight Parents, Gay Children* by Robert A. Bernstein (Da Capo Press, 2003). Liz isn't even certain if they read the books that were sent to them, nor is she sure that they, at her suggestion, attended PFLAG meetings.

In her estimation, Mom and Dad could have done much more to come to terms with her sexual orientation, and they could have done it much sooner. "Their negativity fed on each other as they kept my orientation a secret," she says.

Liz feels that her parents should have talked to others who were open-minded. "Their friends cover the political spectrum, so they could have talked to their more liberal friends and gone online where there are message boards for support."

Hurt that her parents never apologized for all the mud-slinging they did, Liz says, "Coming out as a lesbian in 2015 was the hardest thing I ever did. I knew I was disappointing my parents. But I'm the one who has to go through all the issues of being a lesbian. I have to live daily as a lesbian. They don't!"

Liz found it hard to sympathize with her parents. "What am I supposed to do? Keep this aspect of my life from you?" she wondered.

Parents have to remember, counsels Liz, that their child is not trying to hurt them by coming out. "It's not like I have a drug problem and need to rehab," she adds.

This past year, Liz has been in a serious relationship with a woman. Liz called her parents and told them that if they want to be a part of her life, then they would have to accept her and her significant other. During Christmas, Liz and her partner spent time with Liz's family.

Liz's parents were relieved to see that Liz had made, in their judgment, better choices of lesbian friends than those who her mother regarded as provocative and undesirable in the original camera photos from 2012. They became fond of her girlfriend, so much so that Liz's mother now texts her girlfriend and shares Facebook posts with her.

Since Mom and Dad have become more open, they have not encountered any backlash from telling others that their daughter is a lesbian. While it may have seemed like an inde-terminately long time for Liz's parents to come around, like most parents, their love for their child trumped their fears and eventually led them to accept their child's true self. With this important acknowledgment, Liz finds it easier to accept the truth about herself as well.

Just as denial is a common reaction to finding out your child is gay, so is guilt: *What have I done? How did I cause this? It's all my fault.*

As you will read in the next chapter, parents are not responsible for making their children gay. Dr. Tobkes, in "The Doctor Is In," will clear up these myths as well as others. He will also offer tips on how to resolve guilty feeling many straight parents may harbor.

THE DOCTOR IS IN

Are you experiencing denial? If you agree with any of these statements, then you are probably struggling with denial:

1. My son cannot be gay because he's captain of the football team.
2. My daughter is not a lesbian because she puts on makeup and prefers to wear skirts.
3. My son is not gay because he's had so many girlfriends.
4. My child cannot be gay because my husband and I have been the perfect role models of a heterosexual relationship.

Denial is a defense mechanism used by individuals in order to cope with a reality that is perceived as threatening or damaging to one's self-image or concept of the world. Defense mechanisms are not always pathological but, in fact, are frequently utilized by healthy people in order to adapt to the sometimes unpleasant or disturbing experiences and emotions encountered in life. Defense mechanisms become dysfunctional when they distort one's perception of reality so greatly that they impede emotional growth or impair relationships and daily functioning. In the face of a trauma, such as sudden death of a loved one or a recently diagnosed illness, denial is invoked in an adaptive way to minimize the emotional impact of a situation that is far too uncomfortable to bear. The mature mind, however, will ultimately work past the denial and when better able to tolerate the distressing sentiment, will arrive at the ultimate endpoint of acceptance as part of the "working-through" process.

Denial is the most common defensive reaction that parents experience when first confronted with information suggesting that a child may be gay. This is neither a surprising nor dysfunctional instinct because the vast majority of parents do not have the expectation or wish that their child will be gay. Therefore, they utilize denial in order to cope with a reality that may be perceived as a threat to their self-image or concept of the world.

Upon finding out that a child is gay, many parents are unable to assimilate this new data into their previously constructed notion of their child's identity and future life plan. They are unable to reconcile their child's homosexuality with heterosexual notions that have probably existed in their minds since conception. It is at this point that a parent will utilize denial in order to reject this discordant information and minimize the distress engendered by the reality of having a gay child. Your first reaction may have been something along the lines of "You're not gay. That doesn't make sense. How can you be sure? This is just a phase you will outgrow."

The process of working through your own feelings begins by confronting and breaking down your denial. I have found in my practice that the process of working through denial varies widely from one person to another. There is no "right" way to accomplish this, but there are several avenues that can be taken to successfully identify and deconstruct denial and thereby accept the reality of having a gay child.

It might be helpful for you, as a parent, to begin seeing an individual psychotherapist who can help you better understand the nature of your reaction and help you put this major life event in the larger context of your prior life experiences. This may be a good opportunity for you to take some time to learn more about your own tendencies and to work on improving yourself and your coping mechanisms. As a psychotherapist, I have found that insight is the most crucial ingredient needed to effect change. Without the knowledge and understanding that one is utilizing denial, it is impossible to begin the process of breaking down the defense mechanism and ultimately coming to terms with the reality of the situation.

You may consider starting couples therapy or family therapy, depending on the magnitude of the effect that this new information is having on your relationship with your partner or family. Often in marriages, one spouse is more accepting of their child's homosexuality than the other, which creates tension in the relationship. I have found that in many cases, the same-sex parent has a harder time accepting and internalizing the concept and is, therefore, more likely to turn to denial when faced with the notion of having a gay child. This may be because the parent is over-identified with his or her child and feels the need to call his or her own masculinity or femininity into question. Regardless of the reason, it is fairly common for parents to experience different trajectories of acceptance, which thereby introduces a new marital conflict or exacerbates already existing tension. In some families, the gay child's siblings may not be in denial, and, in fact, a sibling may be the one to introduce the possibility that your other child is gay. Your children can be your greatest source of support and information. I have worked with many parents who have, for the first time in their lives, experienced a role reversal as they sought comfort and reassurance from their (in some cases, very young) child who was able to provide a more enlightened and flexible perspective on the situation.

I have found that a very important factor that determines the ease with which parents are able to work through their denial is the nature of their preexisting relationship with their child. Do you routinely speak about topics of emotional import with your children, or have you avoided such topics until now? If you do not routinely discuss weighty or personally charged topics with your child, it will probably be difficult to start doing so if this particular issue is the inaugural conversation. It might be helpful to meet with a family therapist, if only for a few sessions, just to break the ice and work past the pattern of avoidance. A therapist can help by providing you with the language to express your thoughts and feelings better as well as by imparting tools that foster empathy and understanding.

Friends or relatives who have been through this process with their own child can be an excellent resource. Schedule a time to meet with them to hear about and learn from their experiences. Ask them what they wish they had done differently and what was most helpful for them when they were coming to terms with this same situation. See if you can identify coping strategies that might help you during this potentially difficult adjustment period. Just as there are certain character traits that determine how an individual will cope with a trauma, I believe that there are characteristics that can predict how one will respond to other life surprises such as finding out that a child is gay. Some of these qualities include resilience, ego strength, and flexibility in thinking. If you have bounced back relatively quickly from other life events that you experienced as being adverse, then it is quite likely that after a discrete period of self-reflection and adjustment, you will emerge stronger and better equipped to cope than before. Most parents with whom I have worked have felt that the experience of having a child come out as gay served to strengthen and deepen their relationship. If possible, you should seek out parents further along in the process than you are so you can rest assured that you and your child may grow even closer throughout this pivotal time in his life.

If you cannot think of anyone who has been through the experience of having a child come out as gay, you should seek out open-minded and caring friends or family members who have been supportive and helpful to you during stressful times in the past. When you are feeling vulnerable, it is important to turn to people who will support you without the fear that sensitive information will be shared with others against your wishes. This is even more crucial for those parenting alone. This may be the first "crisis" that you are facing as a single parent, and it will probably be tough to weather these very difficult emotions without the support of a close confidante.

Another factor that will determine how quickly you will overcome your denial is your baseline notion of what it means to be gay. What is the nature of the exposure you have had to gay people? Was your main concept of what it means to be gay culled from watching a few episodes of *Glee* and reading conservative anti-gay marriage propaganda, or do you have regular contact with a gay coworker or family friend? If you have an accurate and realistic idea of what your child's life can be like, you are at a better starting point than someone who is overly reliant on stereotypes and misconceptions. Information is power. Some parents have no gay friends or acquaintances and, therefore, rely on stereotypes or distorted preconceived notions for their information on homosexuality. In my practice, I have noticed that parents feel better when they realize that they are not alone and that there are people like them who are experiencing similar thoughts, feelings, and reactions to having a gay child. There are support groups in the community that you should explore. I would suggest contacting your local PFLAG organization and attending a meeting.

Although denial is a defense mechanism that can sometimes be healthy and adaptive, when facing the realization that your child is gay, denial is only a hindrance in beginning the process of acceptance. The most important steps for working through your denial involve having direct and honest conversations with your child and other family members, reaching out to friends and community supports for additional guidance, and in certain cases, seeking help from a trained professional.

GUILT TO INNOCENCE

"Guilt is not a response to anger, it is a response to one's own actions or lack of action. If it leads to change, then it can be useful, since it is then no longer guilt, but the beginning of knowledge."

—American poet Audre Lorde (1934–1992)

S LICE-OF-LIFE WRITER Erma Bombeck once quipped, "Guilt is the gift that keeps on giving." As far as I'm concerned, there's a kernel of truth in her philosophy. In our society, parents—and especially mothers—believe they have total control of their kids' actions. Therefore, if the children don't behave as expected, you must be a bad parent; consequently, you feel guilty and blame yourself.

I can remember feeling guilty when I discovered my son was gay. I wondered, did I push him to this orientation? Should I have not sent him to local arts camp when he was five? Maybe basketball camp for two weeks would have been better?

Or, would it have been better if I hadn't taken him to Broadway plays such as *Tommy* or *Les Misérables* on weekends when he could have been watching sports games with his dad or friends? Should I have put my foot down when he set his younger sister's hair after she got the dressing table she wanted for Christmas?

But in hindsight, I shouldn't have been in a *mea culpa* state. It was totally unnecessary! I no longer believe, as I was taught, that being gay is a consequence of an overbearing mother with a too-close relationship with her child and a milquetoast distant father.

While views on the origins of homosexuality remain split (nature versus nurture or combination thereof), in a May 2014 Gallup poll, 47 percent of Americans believed that homosexual orientation is present at birth and not environmentally acquired. While conservatives argue that being gay is a *choice of lifestyle*, new research supports the fact that human beings may be inherently oriented toward homosexuality or heterosexuality.

Emotional Journey Toward "New Normal"

Despite the growing body of scientific research pointing to a "gay gene," many parents blame themselves for their child's sexual orientation. Statistically, being gay makes their child a minority, and even with the great strides made toward acceptance, U.S. history has proven that, with every advancement in civil rights, you can expect a backlash against minority groups.

If a parent thinks he can keep a child from being a minority, he will regard her sexual orientation as a "lifestyle," and one she can change. However, as you will see in the stories below, once a parent realizes that the child's identity is not going to go away, and he has to deal with his child's gayness, over a period of time, he will learn to accept and understand the child's sexual orientation.

Straight mother Shawne Duperon thought homosexuality was a lifestyle until she educated herself and began doubting the beliefs of her Baptist faith.

Shawne Duperon, Mother, Fifty

Shawne Duperon, a six-time Emmy-winning media coach and trainer communications expert from Detroit, couldn't believe her ears when she found out through a long-distance phone call that her son James, a high school wrestler, was gay. She was on the phone with her son, who was attending a boarding school in France, and overheard him talking romantically to another boy. Dying to know, she, guileless, asked him, "Are you gay?" to which he replied, "Yes!"

Her bright son, fourteen at the time, never seemed so far away, and it wasn't just because his school was across the ocean. Finding it hard to acclimate to the news, Shawne took his coming out "as a personal attack." Her mind raced with questions: "What have I done to cause this? Maybe I didn't love him enough. Maybe I should have shielded him less from his father [from whom she is divorced]. How can I *fix* this problem? After all, gay people *are* flawed."

Shawne Duperon, who has a doctorate in Communications and Gossip, has spent years observing the ways people convey information, but found herself almost tongue-tied when she had to address her son who admitted he was gay. "It takes guts to look at your collective belief system," she says. Shawne was brought up in the Baptist faith. "I've had to look at myself and my stereotypical perceptions of people," she admits.

Shawne believes that this has been a five-year journey of self-discovery for her and that she has had to face her judgments about minority groups, not just gays. She had to upend her hardwired notions. It has been a road of ups and downs, with progress made toward acceptance, only to backpedal into doubts. But today, she and James, who now works on movie set productions in gay-friendly Los Angeles, have a close relationship that many of James's friends, whose parents are nonaccepting, wish they could mimic.

How did Shawne learn acceptance? Besides a supportive second husband and therapy, she talked to her son about his life within the gay community for a better understanding of his life. She wanted to educate herself.

Shawne believes that parents should be gentle with themselves. Some parents take longer than others to come to acceptance, if at all. You can't force feelings to disappear. But if parents are distressed, she counsels, they should not confide that feeling to their child. Confiding makes the child a codependent—he begins to feel as if he has take care of *you, the parent*!

Many parents, in theory, think being gay should be socially acceptable. However, when the issue affects them directly, it can wreak havoc on an otherwise liberal adult.

Barbara Goldfarb, Mother, Sixty-Seven

"Not in my backyard" is what Barbara thought when her son, Jerry, then twenty-four, came out to her. Although she was a psychoanalyst in a wealthy Fairfield County, Connecticut, town and came from a liberal family in Cincinnati, she was not ready for this.

"I had a knee-jerk reaction," she exclaimed. She thought, "What have I done"—a phrase that continuously played over and over again in her head—"to produce a gay kid?" After all, his *twin* was heterosexual, as was his older brother—both married with children. She had assumed that twin brothers would both be heterosexual.

Looking back, Barbara felt that she should have seen the clues: the fact that her son dated at Middlebury College, but it was always platonic, unlike her other children. One so-called girlfriend has since declared herself a lesbian. Jerry's best friend at the competitive Scarsdale High School was an out gay man.

Barbara noticed that Jerry was always full of "angst" in college, but she excused his temperament because he was "driven." High achieving, he graduated with top honors from medical school.

Before Jerry attended medical school, his mother asked him, "Don't you want to marry a Jewish girl?" While earning a master's degree in medical science from Boston University, Jerry lived in a gay neighborhood in Boston but concealed his orientation, except to a few close friends. "I knew he struggled and probably covered up. I should have been a container for his emotions," said Barbara remorsefully.

Jerry's brothers and his father, a retired operations manager at a teaching hospital, helped her change her outlook from guilty to one where she saw Jerry as the same child she had always loved and admired. Although reluctant at first to divulge to anyone about Jerry being gay, she eventually told her good friends. It is not uncommon for a parent to enter the closet when their child comes out of it. However, Barbara had, after a year, reached the turning point where she told everyone that her son had been married to a nice man since 2011. Jerry lives in Massachusetts, which was the first U.S. state to have marriage equality, and works as a medical oncologist.

Gay kids, like Jerry, not only worry about disappointing their straight parents' dreams for them, but as in J. S. Koppel's case below, about ruining his father's career in the public eye. J. S. would have come out sooner had he not been concerned about embarrassing his father should his son's sexual orientation be leaked.

J. S. Koppel, Son, Forty-Three

A third-generation Birmingham, Alabama, son, J. S. realized he was *different* when he was a teenager at his high school, but he didn't want to reveal his difference to his parents. His father, an attorney, was from the 6th Congressional District of Alabama, and J. S. felt that if he came out, the disclosure, if it circulated, might hurt his father's career. When they moved to Washington when J. S. was fourteen, he continued to worry about affecting his father's political career. "What I knew about [being] gay was cartoonish. Gay people got AIDS in the mid-eighties. It was a foreign concept to me."

J. S. divulged that he was attracted to girls but had "more explicit thoughts" about boys in his head. Because his friends did not think of J. S. as a guy after "chicks," his friends avoided locker room conversation with him. Still, he was not teased in school, nor was he picked last for sports.

Instead of going on double dates with girls, he concentrated on academics, which earned him a freshman spot at Yale University. He spent his spare time reading. Friends were suspicious that he might be gay, but they didn't harass him. After graduation from high school, his senior class went to Rehoboth Beach to party. His two best friends took him to a gay nightclub, where he danced with some gay men. It caused fear inside him. Was this what the future held for him? Not knowing how to proceed worried him.

At Yale, he tried to date a girl for six weeks. It was a chaste relationship that didn't work out. Later that spring, he began a secret affair with a fellow male student that lasted for one-and-a-half years. He finally felt compelled to tell his parents because he was living with his lover in an apartment in Alabama.

His father took it well and told his son in a calm voice that he loved him. His mother was very emotional. You would not have expected this from an otherwise sophisticated liberal who had taught art history at Washington, D.C.'s American University after studying in New York. She was crying and, between sobs, told J. S. that she was sorry that she *failed* him. She felt as if she should have helped him deal with his sexual orientation, but she was "in the dark."

Concerned that J. S. might be unhappy, she wanted him to see a friend of hers in Washington, a psychoanalyst whose specialty was counseling Catholic priests. It didn't seem like a match for a Reform Jew, but J. S. conceded. He had never been to a therapist, but he found his mother's friend easy to talk to. The therapist's report to his mother was that J. S. was well adjusted and fine with being gay. This good news put the Koppels at ease.

J. S. affirms that his parents were wonderful and never pressured him to date. Today, he is married to a man who has a nursing-teaching job at New York University, and J. S. divides his time practicing architecture in Alabama—which was slow to have marriage equality until the SCOTUS ruling in June 2015 that legalized gay marriage in every U.S. state—and in New York.

Like J. S., Andrew Rogers was reluctant to tell his parents he was gay. However, he didn't expect the negative reaction he received to last as long as it did. He is going to come out again in a better setting after having rescinded his first outing. Here's his unique story.

Andrew Rogers, Son, Twenty-Four

Guilt disappoints. While technically, you cannot make a person feel guilty, your expectations for his behavior can make him feel as if he has let you down.

Andrew Rogers should be every parent's dream child. Growing up in Indiana, he took advanced placement courses in high school, where he also was on the soccer, tennis, and cross-country teams. He participated in theater, and in his spare time, he worked at an American Eagle Outfitters clothing store. He didn't date in high school and never got into trouble. He won a partial scholarship to a college within the state of Indiana.

His father, a computer consultant originally from Illinois, and his mother, a hairdresser from Indianapolis, pushed Andrew to succeed. He has an older married sister, but he was the "apple of his parents' eye" until that Sunday after Thanksgiving when his parents drove him back to college and he announced that he was gay at age nineteen.

Dad and Mom were shocked. At first, they asked the questions that many straight parents pose: "Are you sure?" and "How would you know?" Andrew answered with one-syllable answers: "Yes, no." Both were silent; then the questions would start all over again.

Andrew expected them to be shocked, although he says he knew at age seven that he was *different*. Ritch Savin-Williams, author of *The New Gay Teenager* (Harvard University Press, 2006) and Director of the Cornell University Sex and Gender Lab, reports that the average age for a male knowing he's gay is ten.

However, Andrew didn't expect the reaction he received. He was hoping for unconditional love. Instead, he received angry calls and e-mails from his parents saying his soul would be endangered and he would go to hell. He would be banished from society, religion, and school. Andrew's mother was Catholic, but now she's Lutheran. They presented him with religious articles and biblical passages to bolster their point of view. They called their priest. They suggested conversion therapy. Conversion/reparative or "fix-gay therapy" doesn't work. It only makes the gay person depressed, sometimes suicidal, and if employed, only represses homosexual urges for a short time. Because of its horrific side effects, it has been outlawed in California, District of Columbia, New Jersey, and Oregon.

While Andrew worked at home during school vacations, his parents never gave up trying to convert him. When he was at college, he participated in a LGBT club, a social justice club, and campus leader clubs. His father, a smoker, was stressed out over Andrew's identity, which he considered a disorder. His mother warned that if "Dad has a heart attack, it's because of *you*!"

Andrew threatened not to come home if his father continued to yell at him. Dad threatened to not pay for college, to which Andrew replied, "I can't afford to come home then." Now enrolled in a Masters of Health program at Indiana University while a full-time staff member in the School of Education, Andrew finally has given up on his parents. Although all states now have same-sex marriage, his mother is told by customers that if she uses scissors to cut hair on a gay person, they should be thrown away afterward.

"My parents act as if I wasn't their kid anymore. All the good I've done—the awards I received suddenly disappeared. Here I held this deep secret for at least fourteen years. I wish my parents would have seen me as a scared teenager, not a 'fag.' Although parents may feel shame, fear, and anger, so does the child. We have to see each other's perspective and be in the other's shoes—no matter how hard that is. I'm doing everything under the sun for my parents to even acknowledge you can be gay and be a leader and accomplish great things."

Despite the fact that he e-mailed his parents "This is who I am" five years ago, Andrew felt a compulsion last summer to lie to them and say he was straight and that he had been mistaken about being gay. Tired of his parents' recriminations, and his cover-up stories to protect himself from their disapproval, Andrew made that decision, which has resulted in, as he anticipated, his parents treating him differently because he is living the fantasy they had for him. All of a sudden, they are kind and non-threatening. Since that pronouncement, everything has been "hunky-dory."

"It's as if they had amnesia about the whole subject."

The Second Coming Out

As part of the charade, Andrew hides the fact that he is living and in a relationship with another man, who is accepted by his own parents. Andrew may spend Christmas with his parents, but he also visits his boyfriend's parents on the sly in Las Vegas for the rest of the holidays.

Fed up with the exhausting ruse, he is planning a second coming out. What will be different this time? Says Andrew, "I was selfish and didn't think of their perspective at the time. I should have said initially that 'this is really hard for you.'"

Andrew suggests that you make it clear to parents when you come out that it takes time to get over issues such as denial, anger, fear, shame, loss, and guilt. He also thinks it's a good idea to come out in a place where they are comfortable, such as their home, and not in an unfamiliar place like a dorm room. If they become angry, then take a time-out. "Just breathe and let them digest the news. Parents shouldn't immediately ask a million questions, or debate, but just listen."

THE DOCTOR IS IN

Are you experiencing guilt? If you agree with any of these statements, then you are probably struggling with guilt:

1. If I had not let him play with dolls as a child, my son would not be gay.
2. I should not have allowed my daughter to play field hockey in school because it caused her to become a lesbian.
3. I wish I had worked only part-time while my children were growing up so I could have ensured that they developed "properly."
4. I regret getting divorced from my spouse because it caused my child to reject heterosexual relationships and become gay.

Guilt is a state of feeling characterized by an internal conflict that develops upon perceiving that we've done something wrong. We experience guilt when we act in some way that goes against our internal moral compass. Like denial, however, guilt can also be a useful tool. It causes us to examine ourselves by reflecting on our actions and underlying motivations. Ultimately, the experience of guilt can result in making better choices and striving to be a better person. In its healthy form, guilt drives us to analyze and change our behavior, particularly when our actions have adversely affected a friend or loved one. However, guilt becomes maladaptive when it is not rational or justified. In such situations, the feeling of guilt can become all-consuming, causing emotional turmoil without a legitimate reason.

An example of unhealthy or neurotic guilt occurs when we set unreasonably high and unattainable standards for ourselves and then feel bad when we are unable to reach them. For example, someone who feels that it is never appropriate to waste time and always feels badly when she isn't maximally productive will be perpetually plagued by guilt because it is virtually impossible never to procrastinate. A person who holds such an elusive expectation will experience frequent guilt, which will erode her self-esteem over time. Another example of neurotic guilt is when a person assumes responsibility for something that happens to someone else that was totally out of his or her control. For example, a grown child may feel inappropriately guilty that his mother developed heart disease because he didn't monitor her diet and make sure that she took her blood pressure pills. It is unreasonable for a child to assume the responsibility of ensuring that his parent always eats healthfully and complies with her medication regimen. Feeling guilty in this situation is dysfunctional and also implies a sense of self-importance that is inaccurate.

After working through their denial, many parents progress to a state of guilt because they feel a sense of responsibility for having a gay child. They think that this outcome occurred as a direct result of some defect or flaw in their parenting style or ability, and they are plagued by thoughts such as "Where did I go wrong?" and "If I only I had . . ." All parents feel guilty at one time or another for some aspect of their parenting or some quality present in their child. For example, a mother may feel guilty that she worked full-time and blame herself for her daughter not getting accepted into the college of her choice (the implication being that had she been home more, she could have ensured that her daughter had worked harder and earned better grades). Similarly, a father may berate himself for not having had more direct conversations with his son about safe sexual practices when he learns that his son impregnated his high school girlfriend. The reality is that all parents are imperfect and, therefore, your goal should not be to be the perfect parent (an ideal construct that does not exist), but rather to be the best parent that you can be to your specific child.

Parental feelings of guilt that develop after learning a child is gay have two implications that are important to identify and examine. Guilt only arises in situations where one feels responsible for a bad or negative outcome. If you are feeling guilty about having a gay child, you need to realize that you are associating homosexuality with something that is inherently undesirable or adverse. Many people do not feel this way, and your child may not either. When I work with parents who are having a hard time making peace with the idea of having a gay child, I spend a few sessions imparting to them that being gay, while not what they were expecting or hoping for their child, is not, by definition, unfavorable. I often help parents identify the origins of their preconceived notions of what it means to be gay, and after a rigorous examination I guide them to the realization that many of their thoughts are quite distorted and inherently false. You should take some time to try to learn more about yourself by reflecting on when and how your ideas about homosexuality became cemented. You don't necessarily have to work with a psychotherapist to do this. Although it often doesn't occur to people to discuss this with their spouse, when they do, it tends to be very illuminating and therapeutic. Frequently, the stress of a child coming out drives a married couple apart; however, this is counterintuitive to me because this a time when you should work together, helping each other learn more about yourselves and coaching each other to be better parents. The most important initial step in overcoming guilt for having a gay child is realizing that the guilt is dysfunctional because in reality your child's life is no worse for being gay.

Second, the presence of guilt is always associated with the perception of responsibility. In this case, parents feel that they have had some hand in determining the sexuality of their child. According to a May 2014 Gallup Values and Beliefs poll, 37 percent of Americans believe that people are gay due to environmental factors, including parenting, while 42 percent feel that people are born gay. There has been a significant evolution in this attitude since the first time this question was posed in 1977, when 56 percent felt homosexuality was environmentally determined and 13 percent that it was inherent. Currently, an increasing percentage of the population holds the belief that sexuality has a very significant heritable component. Homosexuality does not appear to follow the rules of classical Mendelian genetics since there is no single gene but rather, the model of epigenetics, in which the environment, both uterine and postnatal milieus, affects the way in which genes are expressed. Other traits with strong epigenetic contributions are height, weight, and the development of cancer. Some parents with whom I have worked have expressed guilt about passing down genes that may have led their child to become gay. However, the most common manifestation of parental guilt, in my experience, is the concept that some aspect of their parenting resulted in their child developing a same-sex attraction. To date, there is no data that convincingly correlates individual parental qualities or styles of parenting with child sexual orientation. Interestingly, I have never worked with a gay family in which the child blames his parents for his sexual orientation; it's always the other way around.

Regardless, there's no use crying over spilt, unhealthy guilt. Feeling guilty about something that had nothing to do with you and was unavoidable regardless of anything you might have done differently is not a productive use of emotional energy. Instead, take the time to think long and hard about how your actions now may cause you to experience guilt later, especially if you are prone to feeling guilt. I have found that guilt can best be avoided by anticipating how your current choices and behaviors can potentially result in guilty feelings in the future. For example, by rejecting your child's gay identity, you are, in effect, rejecting him. In my experience, children are significantly more traumatized by parental rejection than they are about being gay itself. The gay youth I have counseled spend more time worrying about how their parents and friends will react to them than they do about any other social, political, or religious implication associated with being gay.

Rather than brooding over what you could have done to prevent your child from being gay, I recommend that you contemplate what may happen if you are not supportive of your child during this difficult time of self-discovery. The ongoing Family Acceptance Project at San Francisco State University (web address: http://familyproject.sfsu.edu/sites/sites7.sfsu.edu .familyproject/files/FAP_Family%20Acceptance_JCAPN.pdf e-mail: fap@sfsu.edu) has shown that gay children who are not supported by their parents are at higher risk for truancy, substance abuse, unsafe sexual behavior, depression, and suicide. If you do not accept the reality that your child is gay and absolve yourself from any associated guilt, you may actually be contributing to an adverse outcome in the long run. In fact, an abundance of data demonstrates that a lack of parental support is associated with distress and dysfunction in gay youth, whereas no evidence exists to definitively prove that parenting methods or styles are pivotal in determining a child's sexuality. I have counseled parents who spent years rejecting their gay child and then came to me with extreme guilt, depression, and regret as well a sense of responsibility for the way in which their child's troubled life unfolded. The sooner you free yourself from crippling, irrational guilt, the sooner your family can move forward together in a positive direction. It's never too late to "come around" and support your child. I have worked with some families in which the parents vehemently voiced disdain for their child's sexuality initially but ultimately shifted their perspective and made amends years later.

Here are some examples of what you might want to say to your child, both because it will make her or him feel loved, supported, and accepted and because it will decrease the likelihood of your developing guilt:

- I feel sad that you have been struggling with this for such a long time. I hope you now know that you can always come to me with anything without worrying that I will not accept you.
- The most important thing to me, as your parent, is that you are happy. I want to do anything I can to help you achieve that goal.
- I am and will always be proud of the kind of person you are, and I am most proud of you right now for having the courage to share this with me. I know how difficult this must have been for you.
- I want to be the best parent I possibly can be for you. I hope you will always feel comfortable telling me if there is something you need from me that I am not providing you.

Guilt can be a great masquerader. Conscious feelings of guilt about one thing can sometimes be representative of underlying guilt about something else. For example, when I work with parents of gay adolescents, they almost immediately express guilt for the things they "did" that, they feel, resulted in their child becoming gay, such as not buying enough toy trucks for their son despite the fact that he only showed an interest in dolls. However, upon closer analysis, there are other more significant things, completely unrelated to their child's sexuality, that they either did or didn't do, which may be more deserving of their guilt. Sometimes these things are repressed from consciousness because they are too painful to tolerate, so instead, a parent may focus on less consequential regrets. For example, a parent may perseverate on the fact that she didn't take her daughter shopping enough (and therefore, she is now a lesbian), but a deeper exploration may reveal that she really feels more distressed by the fact that she didn't allow her daughter to pursue her desire to act in the school shows because she felt it would distract from her studies. Regardless of why you are feeling guilty, I find that the period around a child's coming out is often an ideal time for a parent to reflect on the kind of parent he or she has been. If you are feeling regretful about some aspect of your parenting, you should convey this to your child with an apology and explanation. You might say something like, "I'm sorry I wasn't more supportive of your interest in acting and was focused so much on your grades. If I could do it over again, I would have supported all of your interests."

· 3 ·

FEAR TO FEARLESS

"Fear always springs from ignorance."

—American author Ralph Waldo Emerson (1803–1882)

WHILE GUILT CAN influence a positive change in behavior, fear can stop parents or gay children in their tracks so their outlook is arrested, paralyzing. I can remember lying in bed at night and playing what if? Will my son be able to get the job he wants? What do I do if he continues to be bullied in high school? Who do I go to? What if he contracts HIV?

I feared not only for him but also for myself. Who should I tell or not tell about my child's sexual identity? How will I remember whom I have told? Will my friends gossip about our family?

Fear prevents us from moving forward; it motivates us to run from our problems. The straight parents and gay kids in this chapter will tell you how they gained control so their initial constant worries didn't continue to plague and rerecord in their minds.

Self-knowledge gave the following interviewees the wisdom to overcome their fear and demonstrate to others their truth that they can no longer hide. One such gutsy man is Nasir Fleming.

Nasir Fleming, Son, Nineteen

On the surface, Nasir Fleming, a gay black man, would appear fearless. On May 23, 2014, he was selected as Prom *Queen* at Danbury High School. Popular, smart, and talented, his high school lauded him. He captured his experience in a popular YouTube video that received over 78,000 views, which was picked up and replayed by local news stations.

But not everyone cottoned to him. To some commenters on YouTube, he really pushed the envelope. When Nasir was swanning in his tiara, some people in the gay community thought he was reinforcing negative stereotypes: the gay, swishy, over-the-top, "feminine" man. Others thought it was a mockery of the prom tradition.

Some of the online insults that incensed Nasir the most were reactions to his video posted by forty-five-year-olds. "Parents are usually the ones to blame for discrimination, not the kids," commented Nasir.

However, despite knowing that he might be ridiculed, Nasir wanted to be Prom Queen, as he wanted to send a message about the absurdity of gender labeling to make a point about being himself. "An action cannot be feminine or masculine, it just is," he said. "Once we move past these simple labels, we can work toward lessening violence and societal pressures and creating self-love and true gender equality."

"It wasn't until high school where I realized being a black, gay man in a macho male society in America is extremely scary. . . . Achieving my goals will be far more difficult than it would for a heterosexual white male."

This attitude was much different than when he originally came out in the sixth grade and was teased. As he put it, "I was sure of myself then because I was naive. I thought I could achieve anything."

Nevertheless, Nasir was afraid to tell his biological mother that he was gay, but she was accepting. His aunt and uncle, who adopted him at age five, initially reacted with a common response: "You are too young to know." But eventually they came around and accepted that he did, in fact, know even then. Now, they tell him not to "tone it down"—dress and affect, that is—and support his effort to be himself, even while facing criticism.

Today, at his college in New York, Nasir continues to push the envelope. A member of the LGBT union there and an annual attendee at the True Colors Conference, the largest LGBT Youth Conference in the United States, Nasir is also a contributor to the *Huffington Post*'s "Gay Voices" section and wrote a piece entitled "I'm an 18-Year-Old-Boy Who Wears Blue Nail Polish—Get Over It."

"I love controversy," affirms Nasir, who wants to have his own television show. "Now I understand why people who act outside of their assigned gender roles can be seen as intimidating or threatening: Because we challenge a system that generally forces us to choose to be one way or another. We break societal norms, and this causes fear." Gender and gender expression are fluid concepts.

Like an out celebrity, by making himself visible and heard—even if in a self-deprecating way—Nasir makes fear subservient to his desire to be an individual with his own identity.

Like Nasir, Emily Bruell had a unique method for coming out to peers and parents.

Emily Bruell, Daughter, Nineteen

Emily Bruell, like Nasir, does not like labels, nor does she like feeling afraid.

Not many people come out at their high school graduation, but Emily, valedictorian at Roaring Folk High School in Carbondale (near Aspen), Colorado, did. (Evan Young, a gay valedictorian in nearby Longmont, Colorado, was barred from giving a commencement address in which he planned to out himself. The difference, it seemed, had to do with the fact that Evan's high school is a Charter Academy and disapproved of homosexuality.)

"I couldn't give a speech about talking about identity and leaving this important part of my identity out," confirmed Emily, who showed her principal, Drew Adams, the speech beforehand. Principal Adams called it "perfect." She also shared it with her school counselor, Krystal Wu, who was active in her school's Gay-Straight Alliance.

But she had not shown her speech to her father, Marc, age fifty-two, a technology administrator, and her mother, Debbie, age fifty, a journalist for *The Sopris Sun* (Carbondale, CO), although she had already come out to them and her younger sister, Renee. They were all accepting from the start. She had also revealed this secret to a few of her close school friends.

Because Emily was introverted, the president of her class, Jackson Hardin, was surprised at her delivery speech that included homemade flash cards with words like *smart*, culminating in an Ace card, *gay*. Bound for Bates College in Maine, a college that celebrates diversity, as a science major, Emily says "I continued being the brand 'smart girl,' and working to fill that identity, and to make sure that nothing contrary to it slipped out."

During that June commencement speech, Emily overcame her fear. "I realize that I am gay, and I was terrified of the stigma that label held." To Emily, labels limit and stigmatize a person. "No single label is big enough to hold an entire person."

Emily suggests that all people, not just gays, give up those labels. Judge a person as human, not a compilation of labels. After her positive speech, Emily rid herself of fears. She received a standing ovation but found negative feedback online from strangers; however, she really didn't care about the latter.

Meagan O'Nan was also nervous about people's reactions to her being gay. However, she realized it was *her problem* to conquer, and she chronicles her fear in her book *Courage: Agreeing to Disagree Is Not Enough* (North MS Acupuncture and Holistic Center, 2014).

Meagan O'Nan, Daughter, Thirty-Two

Some adults dance around fear, but not Meagan, who tackled it head-on. Coming out at age twenty-two, a star basketball and baseball player on an athletic scholarship at Mississippi State, Meagan thought she would find acceptance when she announced to her teammates and parents that she was a lesbian. Instead, she was shunned by the Fellowship of Christian Athletes (FCA) and, even worse, by her parents. "Suddenly, groups of people I had been surrounded and supported by began to attack me and act like all I had been was gone forever," she said.

Meagan felt like a failure because she was gay. While studying to get her master's degree in counseling (which she now has), Meagan had been living with a woman, "Clare" Mallory, in Fort Collins, Colorado. Clare is a daughter of a lesbian, so her parent was accepting of her relationship with Meagan from the start. (As we saw in Chapter 1 with Glennda Testone's family, it is not unusual to have more than one gay family member, no matter how distant.) Meagan and Clare later married in May 2014 in New York. It was a second coming out for Meagan. When I interviewed Meagan about fear, her mother,

Robin, was still having a tough time introducing Clare as Meagan's wife. Perhaps, for Robin, introducing Clare as her daughter's wife would mean the end of the dream she had for Meagan to marry a suitable man and bear grandchildren. With a same-sex wife, you cannot hide the relationship. It's not as if she is a "girlfriend" whom you're trying to pass off as a "friend."

Meagan and Clare moved to Mississippi, a place not noted for being gay friendly, yet Meagan's home state. For instance, Marco McMillan of Clarksdale would have been the first openly gay politician were he not murdered at age thirty-four. Mississippi and Louisiana also have the distinction of being the last states to hold out against same-sex marriage. Yet, despite Mississippi's bad karma, Meagan went home to address her real underlying concerns and fears. She felt "called."

Today, Meagan works at a holistic center where her wife works as an acupuncturist. The center attracts a large lesbian and gay clientele. Meagan also speaks to schools and universities about her journey as a lesbian as an integral part of a nonprofit Live Out Loud's Homecoming Project.

It took her mother at least two years to come around. "What we are really seeking is acceptance of ourselves," writes Meagan in *Courage* that offers a deeper look at overcoming fears when faced with feeling like an outsider because of gender, race, religious affiliation, or sexual preference.

Meagan felt as if her mother and others in the community were saying, "I love you, but . . ." Centuries of cultural shaming and condemnation and conditioning contribute to the hurt that inevitably follows.

Robin, an Episcopal bishop's daughter, wanted to "fix" Meagan at a conversion or pray-the-gay-away camp, but Meagan didn't go. Her mother's priest called being gay a "disability," but they also told Meagan's mother, "You have no idea what Meagan is going through."

You would probably think that Meagan's father, Phil, being a southerner and a Catholic, might have a tougher time accepting Meagan's orientation. In fact, Phil, a used car salesman, had an easier time with his daughter being a lesbian than Robin did. (It's not unusual for an opposite-sex parent to be more accepting, according to Dr. Tobkes—see page 29.) He went to counseling with his wife and Meagan, who sought therapy alone first.

While home, Meagan found that, as a writer, she could effectively communicate with her mother, who also liked to write. So, they communicated about their feelings by letters to each other. "We would never be where we are if we had not all been willing to be honest about where we are on our journey. Dialogue leads to understanding, and understanding and acceptance lead to forgiveness, and forgiveness leads to healing, and healing leads to seeing ourselves in the other."

Meagan, through her work as a life coach, as well as lessons gleaned from therapy, knew she could *not* resolve the elephant in the room by getting angry at her parents. Through her willingness to look at her own life, she found that she was limiting herself.

She found courage in herself, and, through deep thinking and self-analysis, she realized that it was *not* the responsibility of her family to fulfill her. She needed to love herself more and speak from a new place where she doesn't feel "less than." It was her responsibility too. Her greatest epiphany was that living from being a victim and seeing the world against her wouldn't work. She needed to move into an empowered life where she was in control. In other words, she had to turn the pain into self-empowerment.

Rosalie O'Grady, Mother, Eighty

It takes a lot to scare Rosalie O'Grady. Her faith buttresses her.

Some parents have conditional love for their children when they hear what they consider the most dreaded words in the English language: "Mom, I'm gay." Not Rosalie O'Grady, a homemaker, who grew up in Philadelphia, Pennsylvania, and has eight children. Her seventh son, Patrick, never came out to her.

But Rosalie, whose husband is deceased, surmised her son was gay when he was a senior in college. Patrick moved in with two lesbians. His mother thought it was odd that he had a post office box for his mail while in college. She asked Patrick about his sexual orientation, and he affirmed he was gay.

Rosalie recollects that in high school Patrick always had lots of girls around him; he was a desirable date for proms and dances. His temperament was gentle. When he was younger, he played with girls in the neighborhood. She was not shocked that he was gay. Neighborhood parents liked him; he spoke to them, whereas other boys his age avoided conversing with adults. But by the time he graduated from college, he had a boyfriend.

Living in the same neighborhood for fifty-eight years, Rosalie has seen many friends' children profess a similar sexual orientation. "The neighbors and I say, 'There is something in the water,'" she relates. One neighbor, a Presbyterian, reads the Bible all the time and is worried that her lesbian daughter will go to Hell. "I don't believe it," affirms Rosalie. "The Roman Empire had tons of gays. Homosexuality has always been there. It's not going away."

Rosalie believes that not everybody is made male or female. Her daughter, Maura, number three of the O'Grady family, while in the sixth grade took lima beans and a paper towel to school for a class assignment. It was not quite the Mendel experiment, but it gave the teacher an opportunity to talk about XY chromosomes. As a result of that lesson, Maura and Rosalie were convinced that there are "in-between" people.

Despite her laissez-faire attitude toward gender and sexuality, which is similar to her late husband's, Rosalie doesn't believe in marriage for gays. When the Defense of Marriage Act (DOMA) was struck down in 2014, Rosalie was appalled that gays wanted marriage because they wanted to access benefits such as healthcare and tax breaks. To Rosalie, a Catholic, marriage is for procreation.

However, she attended Patrick's wedding to Jonah Nigh in the spring of 2015. Because Patrick lives in New York City, Rosalie has less fear for her son being attacked because of his orientation. "Gays need to be with their own peers. . . . I was treated like the Queen of Sheba in a gay club in downtown Philadelphia that Patrick escorted me to. I was treated to stingers by men older than my son. Everybody was calm. I felt more comfortable in this sports bar than a straight bar where there seemed to be more drunkenness."

Rosalie is turned off by gay parades because of the participation of scantily clad gay men, and feels it is hurting the cause of gay rights. She doesn't like the public displays of affection she saw at the Magnificent Mile in Chicago, Illinois, and in Provincetown, Massachusetts, a gay mecca.

To acquaint his mother with the gay population, Patrick gave his mother the book, *Gay and Lesbian Philadelphia* (Arcadia Publishing, 2002) about famous people who are gay in Philadelphia. As they both were raised in Philadelphia, Patrick felt that the book would resonate with her.

She does not worry about Patrick anymore. He is highly educated, with a master's degree in bioethics from the University of Pennsylvania as well as doctoral degree in bioethics from Loyola University. He has a good job. He is married, teaches English to immigrants at a church, and is godfather to his straight friends' children. Patrick, in her opinion, is where he should be.

J. R. Villari, Son, Twenty-One

Like many transgendered men and women, J. R., born Jennifer Rebecca in Staten Island, New York, felt at a young age that he was mismatched with his body. Although some trans people know at the young age of two or three that they're the "wrong" gender, J. R. knew when he hit puberty.

J. R. was at war with the gender he was assigned at birth: "I used to cringe when I heard the command 'girls in one line, boys in the other.' I was never comfortable in the girls' bathroom. My brother wanted me to change for baseball, and I dragged my heels."

His mother wanted J. R. to wear makeup, and J. R. would take it off. Mama, now fifty, tried to send him to high school with a frilly blouse. In his backpack that he took to school, J. R. packed a change of clothes that wouldn't reveal his torso. "I refused to adhere to a dress code, so I couldn't attend an awards ceremony."

The clothes he preferred were baggy and amorphous, and they earned him the titles "dyke" and "butch" in school, even though he never identified with lesbians. He just wanted to be a man. He straightened his hair, and then, when he drastically cut it off, his mother cried out in distress, "You are a reflection of me!" At a pizzeria when he was fifteen, his mother explained to others who thought J. R. looked like a boy, "She's a *she* who looks like a *he*." It was embarrassing.

Luckily, his high school didn't try to change him. It was

more of an inward feeling, gnawing at him and directing him to change. He was a good student and didn't want to stand out—he didn't join the Gay-Straight Alliance in his school.

About a year later, J. R. found out about the concept of transgender. It saved his life! If he hadn't known about how people like himself can actually transition from female to male, he would have continued to struggle and possibly have committed suicide, he confessed.

Still "the fear of the unknown" caused him to be anxious about the reactions of his loud Italian family of three siblings. Says J. R.: "My family had expectations for me, and being transgender was not one of them. But this feeling of being trapped inside your own body doesn't go away on its own."

As enthusiastic as he was to transition, J. R. had to wait until he was eighteen to receive hormone treatment. He was accepted at an LGBT Center in Philadelphia and was taking hormones when he entered college as a female. (His female roommate was initially a little undone when J. R. told her about his transitioning plans, but she quickly became comfortable with the idea.)

J. R.'s family went through therapy to address their apprehensions: his mother was concerned about how the hormones would affect his body, and his father was worried about how people might view his daughter who was transitioning to becoming a son. Would violence ensue from strangers?

J. R.'s mother called the pediatrician as well other doctors to assuage her fears about his physical health. She did research, as did J. R., about the success of the cross-hormonal treatments.

When J. R.'s dad saw that his new son was accepted by friends, his two sisters, and a younger brother, he started to relax his concerns about the prejudice J. R. might encounter.

During his college years, J. R. was buttressed by his college's LGBT group. Today, J. R. states that "transitioning is the best decision I've ever made." He is happy inside his own skin. "It was a confidence builder for me," he says, "and showed me that I could handle tough situations." He doesn't downplay the physical attributes he has gained, too. J. R. has facial hair and hopes to have a mastectomy ("top surgery") so he can take off his shirt. Yes, he can finally use the boys' bathroom. He has not yet had gender reassignment surgery, as it is very expensive.

Still, not everyone knew about his transformation. When J. R.'s voice began to change, he was asked if he was sick. When he was a summer intern at a software development engineer, he did not tell anyone at that office about his gender identity.

In college, J. R. thrived. He made dean's list and graduated with a BS degree in computer science with a minor in biology. Not only are J. R.'s parents proud of his academic achievements, they also now proudly introduce him as their son.

"My parents have been wonderful," says J. R. It probably took his mother about a year—taking slow but gradual steps—to come to acceptance. She was willing to change her expectations for her daughter Jennifer Rebecca and accept J. R. as a son. She took time to learn and research. Having heard directly from doctors and mental health experts that all would be well, she was able to realize that her son made a well-informed decision to transition.

"She knew not to guilt me and be condescending," says J. R. "Mom avoided saying that her daughter is dead, as all parents should."

David and Marie Douglas, Father and Mother, Forty-Nine and Forty-Six

David and Marie Douglas had more difficulties with fear than Rosalie O'Grady, but their resignation that "this is as good as it gets" was ultimately defeated by their courage to examine their religious upbringings and face their fear head-on.

How does a father, son of a Presbyterian minister and Pentecostal mother, come to terms with his middle son being gay? How did David, who was disillusioned with his church for two to three years, and Marie achieve peace? How did Marie get to the point where she proudly told people at her job as a physician's assistant and school board volunteer that her son is gay?

"I didn't hear anti-gay remarks growing up in the Midwest," says David, now a farmer for a food co-op in Deltona, Florida. "My father was a moderate Libertarian pastor who had four degrees. We always debated at the dining room table."

Later in life, David heard homophobic jokes at his job as a researcher and at church. "Lesbians and gays are not treated well by the church," attests David. Marie, raised as a Baptist but now nondenominational, agrees.

David and Marie are the parents of two boys and a girl. The

middle child, Howard, announced that he was gay at age thir-teen—on Friday, April 14, a date his father will always remember. Although his parents suspected Howard's sexual orientation, they were still shocked to hear the news. Adopted at age seven, Howard had wanted to be a girl since he was two years old. From ages eight to ten, he still wanted to be a girl and stayed away from rough-and-tumble sports. In middle school, he was quiet. He had telltale signs of a stereotypical gay male: a limp wrist and a lisp, characteristics thought to be out-dated and politically incorrect, but still heard in conversations about gays. David asked his son if he was gay and, if so, to rate himself on a "gayness scale" from one to ten. Howard replied that he considered himself a three.

In seventh grade, Howard complained to his parents that he was harassed at least weekly. He became sullen and depressed. Because of the abuse, he completed eighth grade online.

Although Howard's parents were reassuring and told him that they were going to love him no matter what, his only sister, seventeen, outed him against his wishes. The shock sent him back into the closet. Howard told his mother, who has a gay cousin, that he would act straight around her family so she wouldn't have to deal with the "whole gay thing." David told his family in New Jersey but admits that he was numb for a while, probably four or five months, after Howard's confession.

"My health was affected," affirmed David. "I shouldn't have told him that it was the wrong path for him to take and asked him, 'What are you going to say to girls who ask if you're gay?'"

Marie was very emotional and in denial, saying, "I just can't believe it!"

David had real fear. It is a rule in the Douglas family that you cannot date until you are sixteen, at which time you are thought to be mature to make sensible decisions regarding sexual involvement. (See "The Doctor Is In," which addresses this fear as well as others.) Howard told his parents he had a boyfriend. David warned him that condoms can break.

He and his wife worried about people discriminating against Howard at a job. A gay friend of theirs told Howard not to come out at work, at least not initially.

The Douglases ultimately realized that God gave them this child as a blessing. Their child was the same as any other "mainstream" child, only with a different sexual orientation. They realized they were the adults, and Howard was the child trying to figure out his unchartered journey.

David, in particular, did research on gay issues and drew on his relationships with gay friends and colleagues. He lived with two gay men in Jacksonville, Florida, in his thirties, and reached out to them while Howard was in his teens. David came to rely on their observations, such as the fact that Howard was never going to change—he was born gay.

David recommends that parents talk to other parents in the same situation, not judge gay people and not get into theological arguments with others. "I look at the world differently," he says. Howard, who his father says likes to write and is very intellectual, accepts himself. Whenever he has uncertainties, he talks to his parents. The door is always open.

THE DOCTOR IS IN

Are you experiencing fear? If you agree with any of these statements, then you are probably struggling with fear:

1. My gay son will get HIV.
2. My gay or lesbian child will probably become a drug addict or commit suicide due to a more difficult life.
3. My gay or lesbian child will be bullied and/or harassed just as I have seen on the news has happened to other gay and lesbian children.
4. My son will not be able to get a good job in finance because he is gay.

Fear is the feeling of doom or apprehension that plagues someone who senses that something bad is going to happen. From an evolutionary perspective, fear can be quite adaptive. It is the emotion that underlies the fight-or-flight response that for millennia has protected human being from predators and other threats to their survival. The sensation of fear can be what motivates one to take action to protect oneself. However, when present in excess or to an irrational degree, fear can also be crippling by leading to an unhealthy and unproductive repetitive spiral of "what if" thinking. In these situations, often the magnitude of the perceived threat is exaggerated and sometimes based on distorted or dysfunctional thoughts.

Consequently, the fear becomes maladaptive, resulting in a state of functional incapacitation.

When working with patients to address their fears, my approach is usually a two-step process. First, we assess the likelihood of the person's fear actually becoming a reality. And second, if the fear is, in fact, shown to be probable, we work on finding ways in which the feared outcome can be mitigated. I apply this model with parents struggling with fears related to having a gay child.

It is quite common for parents or family members of a gay child to struggle with some degree of fear, especially early on in the process of a child's coming out. While there is certainly an underlying rationality to their fear, I have found that it is the magnitude and perceived loss of control that tend to be the distorted components associated with the fear. In my experience, this fear can have various manifestations and occur in several realms.

Fundamentally, the parents' primary concern is the child's well-being. Many straight parents have a particular bias toward what it means to "live a gay lifestyle," which, for them, conjures up images of drug abuse, sexual promiscuity, and moral corruption. Upon learning that their child is gay, parents may make the mental leap toward a "worst-case scenario" situation and react with a sense of distraught panic as if some apocalyptic, unalterable destiny has been set in motion. In order to demonstrate my two-step approach so that you will be able to put it into practice in your own life, I will review the most common fears parents have voiced to me, analyze the evidence behind them, and then discuss what can be done to minimize the probability of their occurrence.

Health Concerns

The worry that their gay child will contract sexually transmitted diseases (especially HIV or Hepatitis C) as a result of promiscuous sexual activity is almost ubiquitous among heterosexual parents. The statistics are a bit staggering, so it is not surprising that parents are quite alarmed by the risk. Gay and bisexual men are severely afflicted by HIV. According to the Centers for Disease Control and Prevention (CDC), in 2010, gay and bisexual men aged thirteen to twenty-four accounted for 72 percent of new HIV infections among that age demographic. Fortunately, the risk of sexually transmitted diseases can be drastically reduced by taking simple precautions. This is an example of a fear that is not necessarily overestimated; yet it has a fairly easy and straightforward solution. The correct use of a condom for all sexual encounters will decrease the risk of HIV transmission to an infinitesimal level. In addition, the use of pre-exposure prophylaxis (in the form of daily oral antiretroviral medication administration) has been shown to lower the risk of HIV infection by up to 92 percent in sexually active gay men. The medication works by preventing the contraction of HIV in an individual who is exposed to the virus. Many parents are uncomfortable with the idea of their child, gay or straight, having sex, and therefore, they avoid broaching the topic of safe sex. I have found that this avoidance is even more pronounced in straight parents of gay children. Still, it is imperative that you and your child discuss these issues; a conversation about safe sexual practices and education regarding the transmission of sexually transmitted infections (STIs) can be a good place to start. Parents of gay children have told me that since they are not familiar with the particulars of gay sex, they don't feel qualified to engage in such a conversation. My response to them is that even though the specific sexual acts may be different, the precautions that need to be taken are the same as those that straight people should take. Moreover, conveying the message that you care about your child by having the conversation in the first place is just as important and necessary as the content of the safety information. *The message to always use a condom is a crucial, potentially life-saving one that must be delivered.* Beyond this basic lesson, your child should also grasp your warm, unconditional love for him and your unfailing concern for his health and well-being. Self-esteem and the instinct for self-preservation develop as a direct result of feeling loved and cared for by others—most of all, by parents. In my experience, the teenagers who choose not to protect themselves are not necessarily the ones who don't know about the benefits of condoms, but instead are those who do not feel the loving, protective instincts of their parents.

Research has shown that when gay teenagers are rejected by their family, they tend to devalue themselves and, as a result, are less likely to make efforts to protect themselves from HIV. In a sense, it becomes a self-fulfilling prophecy: Parents worry that their child will contract HIV; their fear paralyzes them from accepting the reality of their child's sexual orientation; because the child feels rejected and hopeless, he does not develop a strong sense of self-esteem and a desire to protect himself from disease; ultimately, the child does not take precautions and contracts the virus just as the parents feared from the beginning. Moreover, data supports this. A study done by the Family Acceptance Project shows that rejected gay youth are three times more likely to contract HIV and other sexually transmitted diseases than those who report feeling accepted by their families.

An additional step you could take to ensure your child's safety would be to schedule an appointment with a pediatrician or adolescent medicine physician who has experience in this realm. Setting up such an appointment for your child would send the message that you support him and want to ensure his appropriate medical care and continued good health.

RECAP

Fear: My child will definitely contract HIV and other sexually transmitted diseases because they are rampant in the gay community.

Evaluation: Your fear is backed by evidence. It is true that being gay increases the risk of contracting HIV and other STIs.

Response: Making smart choices with regard to sex—most notably, deciding to always use a condom—will significantly decrease the risk of contracting an STI. The factor that weighs most heavily in determining whether gay teenagers will take such precautions is whether they feel that their life has value, which is a direct manifestation of the sense of love, support, and connectedness they feel from loved ones. *This is something that is very much in your control.* Make it clear that you feel unconditional acceptance of your child, and he will make good choices and be much less likely to jeopardize his health.

Mental Health and Substance Abuse

Many studies have demonstrated the increased risk of drug and alcohol abuse (20 percent to 30 percent of the population) in gay and lesbian adolescents compared to their heterosexual counterparts (9 percent of the population). In many cases, the substance abuse is a form of self-medication, a quick way to ease the shame and pain associated with rejection that often accompanies the coming-out process. In the context of an unsupportive and homophobic environment, gay and lesbian teenagers often escape into substance abuse and other maladaptive behaviors. In addition, it has also been shown that the incidence of psychiatric problems, particularly depression and anxiety, is similarly elevated in gay adolescents.

In my experience, there is a clear correlation between the likelihood of teenagers becoming depressed or anxious and turning to substances and the lack of support from close friends and family members in their coming-out process. One particular study estimated that gay children who were rejected by their family were eight times more likely to attempt suicide, six times more likely to be depressed, and three times more likely to abuse drugs or alcohol than gay children who reported feeling accepted by their families. The best way you can help your child not to feel rejected is by remaining involved in the details of his or her life and by not avoiding topics that may make you uncomfortable. Avoidance of certain areas sends a tacit message that you may not be accepting of these things. *Ask your child how she is feeling on a regular basis.* Coming out often involves multiple steps, and the best way to support your child is by offering support and interest in the process as a whole. If your child expresses distress or appears to be suffering, make a point of asking her if she would like to speak with a counselor.

RECAP

Fear: My child will become drug addicted and suicidal because he is gay.

Evaluation: Your fear is backed by evidence. There are higher rates of drug and alcohol abuse, depression, and suicide in gay teenagers than in their heterosexual counterparts.

Response: Again, studies have demonstrated that it is the children who feel rejected and isolated from friends and family who tend to turn to drugs and alcohol as a way to numb their pain. *This does not have to be your child.* The way you support and nurture her during her coming out—and for the rest of her life—will significantly reduce the risk of experiencing substance abuse or mental health problems.

General Well-Being

Of all the hate crimes reported annually, 28 percent involve sexual orientation–based violence. Therefore, it's natural that parents of a gay child will have concerns about that child's general well-being. Beyond the fear of physical harm, parents have expressed a wide array of worries, including their child being ridiculed and rejected by peers and experiencing job discrimination. While it is less likely that your child will be physically abused for being gay, it is, unfortunately, quite probable that he will experience some degree of verbal harassment or name calling. Parents of a gay child typically do not have the shared experience of being gay and, therefore, cannot truly relate to the feeling of being in this particular "out group." That said, it doesn't mean that you cannot develop a "radar" for discovering whether this is going on and help your child combat it.

The first obvious step is simply to tell your child that he should come to you right away if anyone is making disparaging comments or threats. Many children, even when told that, remain silent when they are bullied because they feel ashamed or humiliated; they even place the blame on themselves. In addition, they worry that the situation will get worse or the bully will retaliate if confronted. Therefore, it is important that parents be on the lookout for other signs that may indicate that their child is being bullied at school. Such indicators include a sudden resistance to going to school, a decrease in making social plans after school or on the weekends, an unexpected decline in grades, feigning illness to avoid school and other events, and recurrent damage to or loss of property or clothes. If you notice any of these things, you should approach your child in a direct and straightforward manner about your concern for his well-being.

If you confirm that your child is the victim of bullying or harassment, the next step would be to schedule a meeting with the appropriate supervisor (the school principal, camp director, boy scout troop leader, baseball coach, and so forth) to discuss the situation. Most schools have zero-tolerance policies with regard to bullying, and you should ensure that the proper steps are taken to swiftly remedy the situation. You should unconditionally support your child, never minimize the experience or tell him that he is overreacting, and work together to formulate contingency plans to ensure that he is safe. Such a plan should include when to ignore the bully and when to speak up. (It is often empowering and helpful for a child to respond with something direct and clear such as, "Stop!" or "That's not funny.") The plan should also involve routes to take between classes and to and from school to ensure that there are adults in the vicinity at all times.

I have found that the most important prognostic indicator for a child being targeted for his sexuality is having a safe haven retreat at home. A child's resilience to bullying is based on whether he feels that he has the loving and unconditional support of his family, which can serve as an anchor for him. If a child feels judged or ostracized by his family, it is almost impossible to recover from external humiliation.

RECAP

Fear: My child will be discriminated against because of his sexuality.

Evaluate: Your fear is backed by evidence. Although it is far more likely that your child will be the recipient of verbal teasing because of his sexuality, it is, unfortunately, a distinct possibility that, at some point, he will also be physically assaulted for being gay.

Response: The best way to prevent this from becoming a problem is early identification. Generally, I have found that the situations that become violent are the ones that escalate over time without outside intervention. You should ensure that your child feels like home is a safe place where he can tell you anything without fear of judgment or ridicule. If your child reports a situation in which he is being teased or bullied, you should assess the magnitude of the situation and involve the supervising adult in the environment where the harassment is occurring. In addition, you should help your child develop a means of responding to such attacks so he feels confident and prepared to handle ridicule.

In summary, some things that you might want to say to your child, both because it will make him or her feel loved, supported, and accepted and because it will help you address your fears are:

- I am so happy that you feel comfortable enough to talk to me about being gay. I want you always to feel like you can talk to me about any aspect of your life without worrying that I will judge you. I love you very much, and that is always what matters most.

- I cannot emphasize enough how important it is to protect yourself and your partner by always using condoms when having sex. Your physical health is incredibly important to me, and I want to make sure that you are doing everything in your power to preserve it.

- If you ever feel that you are being victimized or bullied because of your sexuality or any reason whatsoever, please let me know so we can come up with a plan to ensure that it does not continue. I will always be here to protect you and ensure your well-being.

- We are so proud of the person you have become and that you are part of our family.

ANGER TO CALM

"No man can think clearly when his fists are clenched."

—American drama critic George Jean Nathan (1882–1958)

WITH CLENCHED TEETH and a painted-on smile, as if to say, "Everything is okay," I held on to anger, resentment, and a "poor-me" attitude: This was my modus operandi for a year as I tried to hide my anger. Long story short: It didn't work in the long-term. As we've seen in the previous chapters, emotions such as fear and guilt can bleed at the edge into other emotions such as anger.

I didn't want others to know about our family's secret, but it was hard to keep up appearances. I avoided people in case they asked me questions. I was in a swirl of private guilt, but felt I should obligate the public. Matters of family, gender, and culture stirred together into a fiery-flavored stew.

Anger is an uncomfortable feeling. It causes you to react, not act. It is not a good foundation for decision-making. Your child's future is unclear, and with it, so is yours. Will you be accepted and respected as you were before in your town? Just the fact that you now have to worry about your standing as well as hers or his, through no fault of your own, is enough to make you angry.

"Why me?" "Why do I have to go through this?" "What have I done to deserve this?" plays over and over in your head. You think that you are a victim, and even unconsciously you may begin to feel indignant that this situation has been forced on you.

As you will read in the following stories, unresolved anger about sexual orientation can and will lead to estrangement between a parent and a gay child. The anger can get displaced onto the child, the husband, the sibling, the office. Some gay and lesbian children would rather leave their homes than be at home and suffer their parents' wrath.

Brad Kukakos, Son, Thirty-Four

Brad Kukakos grew up in Ohio, near Wheeling, West Virginia, where the coal mines were shuttered in the 1980s by the Environmental Protection Agency, leaving many of the town's citizens out of work. His father, a former coal miner, now seventy-two, relied on odd jobs as a roofer and landscaper to get by, as well as alcohol and welfare payments. His mother worked as a secretary at a bottle cap factory.

The youngest of four, Brad tried to make things better for his family. He was particularly close to his mother. If friends were coming over to their habitually messy house, it was always Brad who cleaned it up beforehand.

Yet, he was depressed. Acting out his self-disgust in junior high and high school, he kept his head down. He knew he was gay at age eleven, but he also was aware that neither the townspeople nor his family would approve. "It was all white, with no diversity," he said. In small-town Ohio, kids used to play games in high school like "smear the queer," after all. Still, despite the overt prejudice and his own shame, Brad had an active, successful life in high school: friends, a passion for sci-fi, and practices with the high school marching band.

Although his hometown now has a few gay people, while he was growing up, they were regarded as "sick, awful, drug addicts, even child molesters," and as a result no one Brad knew was out. In those days, *Will and Grace* had not been invented, but *Richard Simmons* and MTV's *Real World* were on television and became Brad's entrée into the gay world.

"As a kid I wanted a Barbie, but of course, never got one. I told my siblings I was gay when I was a sophomore in college at Ohio U. in Athens, Ohio. My sister who still lives in Ohio blabbed it to everyone in the family, including aunts and grandma." One, his aunt Tracy, who never had kids, told him, "I love you no matter what."

Brad never had a conversation with his father about being gay. Luckily for Brad, his father was perfectly content living vicariously through his two other sons, taking delight in hearing about their sexual conquests of "chicks."

When I interviewed Brad, his sister, who had four children, would not let him see her kids because she thought he would molest them or convert them to being gay. She believed that being gay was a choice and lifestyle, as does Brad's Ohio brother. (One wonders whether she has changed her mind, given that Ohio has since elected State Senator Rob Portman, who has a gay son and has come out in favor of marriage equality.)

Brad did encounter harassment at college, even though he was in a gay support group. When spotted holding hands with a boyfriend, he was called a fag. When he brought his boyfriend home from college, his mother became upset when Brad referred to his partner endearingly as "Sweetie" and "Honey."

As Brad's mother became more religious in her Methodist faith, she repulsed Brad by saying she was praying for him and he needed to come to Jesus so he wouldn't burn in hell for eternity. Finally, years of prejudice and repressed inner turmoil caused him to explode like a volcano. He told his mother to "take her religion and shove it." He didn't want to be dragged into unhealthy places and finally decided to stop accommodating her. Brad distanced himself from his mother.

Brad's advice to parents is "stop with the church stuff." Promising to pray for a son or daughter's sins will only alienate him or her. Don't preach. Let the child have his or her own say and find out how to feel about being gay.

Sometimes, it's easier to move away than be in constant conflict with a family that lacks understanding or is openly hostile. Brad moved to Columbus, Ohio, where he knew four people from his hometown. Later, he moved farther away, to Chicago, Illinois, for eight years. Finally he moved completely out of the region and has settled for good in sunny Los Angeles, where he works in information technology.

Mom finally came around, due to conversations with a gay older cousin who takes her to football games and mows her lawn. Somehow, just knowing a gay person can help you familiarize yourself with her or his perspective and can help you change your outlook about the gay community.

Once a year, Brad goes back to his hometown to see his family. His mother, in particular, is more accepting.

Derek Moreno, Son, Forty-One

Derek Moreno grew up in Las Vegas, Nevada, the son of a Hispanic grocer whose Caucasian wife worked in the same grocery store. His father referred to his gay son as "little fruit." His sister, five years younger, and cousin, Connie, also lived with them, and his father referred to Derek as one of "the girls." Derek was physically small and reached puberty late.

Defying his slow maturity, the "little fruit" turned out to be a Big Man on Campus. Derek came out to his friends first at age sixteen, then his parents when they were about to get divorced.

Because he received good grades in high school, was in with the "cool kids," and involved in high school theater, which had a healthy blend of gay and straight dramatists, Derek was not teased. He was a drum major, contributed to the school newspaper, and was acknowledged for his efforts at school, but not by his father, who was often out of control, drinking too much, and frequently erupting into bouts of anger directed at his family. To this day, Derek doesn't like to be alone with his tempestuous father.

However, in middle school, before he hit puberty and came

into his own, he was teased. Other kids picked on him because he was not athletic and was considered "girly," with an undeveloped body and a high-pitched voice. In gym class, he was afraid to change clothes and shower for fear of being teased. Derek never wanted a girlfriend and knew in Cub Scouts and elementary school that he was gay. Campouts and sleepovers made him nervous.

On his own, Derek went to a born-again Christian church that his friends attended. It was the worst place he could be. Although Derek didn't want people to know he was gay, the church must have sensed it, as its congregants tried to convert him. If he identified as straight, they said, he wouldn't go to hell. But Derek couldn't change. If he kissed a boy, he would feel guilty afterward, as he remembered the church's doctrine, but his guilt didn't prevent him from wanting to kiss members of the same sex again and again. Guilty and angry, he quit church. He was not in need of reparative therapy or "pray the gay away."

One person who was always had his back was his mother. After Derek came out, she told others that her son was gay and went to the library to educate herself about what to expect when a family member is gay.

Like his mother, Derek doesn't think parents should categorize gays, trying to ascribe a "one size fits all" solution to every gay man's and woman's unique problems. They should be looked at as individuals without labels.

After high school, Derek found his niche dressing live dancers in Las Vegas drag shows. As a member of the Theatrical

Wardrobe Union, he has been in New York for sixteen years now and supervises a costume wardrobe department. He sews, fits actors, dresses actors backstage, and calls the theater "home"—a place where he can be himself. (He says that the television and film industry is more closeted.) When not backstage, he spends time on the West Coast, because his partner of fifteen years is a dancer and director there. Despite Derek's accomplishments in his profession and his good grades in high school, he still has not gained acceptance from his father, the only one in the family who does not approve of his sexual orientation. Derek feels unloved by his macho father. This rejection makes Derek angry. He won't allow himself to be alone with his father, who still drinks to excess and becomes out of control with insults directed at his son.

Kelly Small, Daughter, Twenty-Five

Kelly Small didn't come out to her parents until just recently. She was, as she put it, "half out to her straight friends," who she said knew already. Although she didn't have a girlfriend until she was twenty, she affirmed that she knew she was a lesbian when she was twelve.

Good at softball, her best friends in high school were boys. "I didn't want to be super-butch," she says. "My mother used to hide my baggy clothes in the laundry." She is a lipstick lesbian (a lesbian known for wearing makeup) and is often mistaken for a heterosexual woman by men who hit on her.

Kelly's "Irish twin" brother is fine with her being a lesbian. However, her parents are not—which makes her angry. "It was a bloodbath," states Kelly, whose Catholic father didn't talk to her for a month after she came out. Her mother, a devout Lutheran, threw a Bible at her head and told her to take an anti-gay pill. Hardly accepting of her parents' shortcomings, Kelly is just angry that her mother makes comments like, "Well, at least your brother got it right. He's getting married." This kind of verbal bashing infuriates her.

Even though she dated a girl her last year-and-a-half in college, her parents' homophobia pushed her back in the closet for almost two years. Most of her friends are straight.

Seeing her parents' reactions to her father's gay brother initially kept Kelly quiet about her orientation. "I was terrified of being gay. . . . I have a house with a straight roommate [whom her mother believes Kelly is dating], but frequent a gay section of Chicago called 'Boys Town,'" she says. "I was initially scared to be associated with Boys Town for fear everyone would know I was gay."

Not only are her parents homophobic, so are her employers. At the male-dominated car company where she works, she hears homophobic remarks. She is the only girl in operations, and men hit on her. Before her current job, she worked in sales for bars and Soldier's Field stadium, where she also heard comments. She has not introduced her girlfriend to her parents, as Kelly wants to protect her.

Kelly keeps trying to get her mother's approval and wishes her mother would take off *her* armor. Kelly used to be "the apple of her parents' eye" and is angry that all the good she has done has seemingly disappeared just because she is a lesbian.

Still, Kelly is making efforts to calm her own anger and deal with adversity in a constructive, not destructive, way. Kelly's friend Eddie has taught her how to live openly as a lesbian and accept herself. She has found a church that accepts her, and she is able to answer insults with clear, confident, non-biased comments—not fury. She has explained to her dad, brothers, and extended family what it feels like to be a lesbian and how it's not a choice. She even brought her brother to an LGBT-exclusive event in Chicago so he can learn about her milieu.

Family is the hardest part. Her father understands. However, Kelly's mother is still angry, as is Kelly, despite all of her best efforts. Kelly can't help but feel exhausted trying to win her mother's acceptance while trying to heal her own bruised emotions at the same time.

Wendy Mandel, Mother, Thirty-Eight

Sometimes the hurricane-like force of anger is so great against a nonaccepting spouse that it climaxes in divorce. This is what happened to Wendy Mandel, a patient specialist and crises call receptionist at a domestic violence shelter, who lives in a suburb near Abilene, Texas.

Wendy said, "Ninety percent of the reason why I left Gary," who she divorced over ten years ago, "is the way he treated Jerry, who is gay." Gary is so critical of their son Jerry, who came out to his mother in eighth grade, that Jerry doesn't want to see his father. Gary insists that maybe Jerry is bisexual, as he cannot stand the thought of him being one hundred percent gay.

Gary, age forty, who his ex-wife dubs a "redneck," is a machinist at a tool-and-die company. Wendy says he has always tried to change Jerry's interests, buying him tractors and macho-type toys. Even Wendy tried to steer her son to more traditionally masculine hobbies at first, but quickly saw it wasn't working.

"I knew Jerry was gay from the time he was three or four," confirmed Wendy. He wanted to be Britney Spears and would dance on the athletic field like Britney. Jerry was obsessed with Barbies and high heels. "He told me he wanted to be a girl at age three."

Teased in middle school, Jerry would respond, "Yeah, I am gay. You'll have to come up with something better than that." At a time when Jerry was in a relationship with a guy that was not going well, Wendy found Jerry to be depressed and argumentative. He didn't want to go to school. His mother took him to a behavioral therapy center and he was put on antidepressive medications, which made him withdrawn. Eventually he was weaned off the meds, and by the time he got to high school, he was "out and proud." Jerry had T-shirts made that read "Straight Against Hate."

Jerry's coming-out letter to his mother said he didn't want her to be disappointed and didn't want her to think it was a "phase" or that he was bisexual. Her reply was "I'll always love you. I don't care if you love purple people."

However, not everyone in Jerry's family is as accepting. His Southern Baptist relatives want to "save him" and insist that he pray for a change in his sexual orientation. Wendy has been told by some family members that she is "grooming" Jerry for the gay lifestyle. His aunt, two years younger than Wendy, disapproves, but they still see each other. Their disagreements, however, are too strong for them to be friends on Facebook.

Despite having some bigoted relatives, Wendy is supported by friends, particularly one gay man who grew up in Texas but now lives in Florida with a partner who attends the gay-friendly Metropolitan Church, and some relatives: her mother, half-brother, aunt, and uncle.

She has made her home a haven where Jerry is heard. "You have to remember that I'm the adult, he's not," she says.

Deborah Leemon, Mother, Fifty-Nine

Deborah's daughter Lane came out at age sixteen. She, now thirty, is married to her partner, and lives in a conservative rural community that won't even publish an ad for PFLAG in the local paper. This hateful atmosphere worries Deborah.

Lane, adopted at age two by her stepfather, had a tough time trying to fit in in high school. Her Episcopal priest told her to be closeted until age twenty-one so she wouldn't be harassed. She became involved with a male drummer in high school. They worked on a variety show on Friday and Saturday evenings. Her mother, an auditor for the healthcare industry, said Lane used to flirt with band members, lost weight, and was trying to attract men.

So, when Lane announced she was a lesbian, her mother was shocked, as Lane's persona seemed to be heavily rooted in heterosexuality. Lane lied to people and said she was straight, hanging out with "the fringe," the so-called Goth kids, in high school. She attended a technical program in cosmetology for dramatic arts while still in high school.

Unhappy, Lane began cutting herself. She wrote a paper in high school that grabbed the attention of her school counselor, who was worried for her safety. Lane was given a psychological test that classified her as depressed. She and her family went to therapy, and Lane claimed that she was not going to fix being gay in the psychologist's office.

Continuing her education, Lane went to the same fundamentalist college that her mother attended. It was the quickest way to finish a degree while working. But at South Nazarene, she encountered homophobia again. This made her mother particularly angry. She did not expect her alma mater to be prejudiced against her daughter.

Although Deborah grieved for the loss of a life she expected for her daughter, she was accepting of her daughter and wife and walked her daughter down the aisle. However, one aspect of Lane's life did make her mother angry: the segregation of her daughter's friends from the straight world.

Deborah doesn't like her daughter associating only with other lesbians. After all, Deborah's blind father raised her with the philosophy that minorities should be mainstreamed. He was head of Handicapped Services for Oklahoma State. As Lane, a recruiter for a technical school, is always angry over injustices, her mother was surprised that she would isolate herself into a minority group.

Katy Bourne, Mother, Fifty-Two

Sometimes, parents are so accepting of their gay children that they can't even imagine any straight parent having qualms. So it is with Katy Bourne, jazz singer and marketing blogger for artists in Seattle.

Katy responded to a blog post I wrote, which was based on findings from the Family Acceptance Project at San Francisco State that purported that most coming-outs do not go well, at least initially. Almost incensed, she responded by saying that I was being negative; there were coming-outs that were empowering and self-affirming. I learned my lesson.

Originally from a "red state" environment in Oklahoma, where she assured me most people did not come out, Katy was proud of her son Edward, age seventeen, when he came out to her and her ex-husband. Edward texted them and said, "I know you both know this already . . ." Not only did Edward think his parents knew he was gay, but his older brother Ethan claims he surmised two years ago that Edward was probably gay because of his interest in *Glee* and the way he carefully coiffed his hair.

Edward was bullied in middle school, where he was perceived as gay or "soft." A good friend turned on Edward instead of supporting him. The school didn't discipline the bully, as none of the administrators or teachers saw the taunting, which was frustrating and upsetting.

Katy called Edward's coming out an example of her son's best qualities: "heightened emotional intelligence, sensitive, and gutsy." She admits that she would never have had the self-confidence at his age to reveal her sexual orientation. "I've always been tolerant and had gay and lesbian discussions with him at a young age." Katy had an inkling that Edward was gay when he wanted to attend the Fall 2010 Seattle Pride Halloween Parade as Lady Gaga. She has attended the parade, in a carriage no less, with him during a recent Seattle Pride.

Edward is in a tolerant high school at Seattle Center. Kids are out in an open environment, so Edward has more friends with whom he is comfortable. It's an accepting liberal environment where Edward is a vocalist, musician, and dramatist.

He and his mother live in an arts community where the gay population is well represented. Katy regularly reads *Huffington Post Gay News*, using the articles as jumping-off points to start discussions with Edward. She voices her concerns about her fears for his future, and he's able to converse freely, knowing that he is loved unconditionally.

THE DOCTOR IS IN

Are you experiencing anger? If you agree with any of these statements, then you're likely struggling with anger:

1. My daughter chose to be a lesbian to get back at me for forcing her to take ballet for all those years.
2. If my wife hadn't focused so much time on her career, our daughter would be straight.
3. I am angry at God for making my son gay.
4. My son shouldn't have spent so much time with his theater club advisor, because the advisor turned him gay.

Anger is a universally understood emotion because it is expressed on a regular basis in a wide variety of contexts. It is characterized by antagonism toward someone or something that is perceived as deliberately having done you wrong in some way. When present in excess or in an uncontrollable fashion, anger can be quite destructive and unproductive. It can lead to emotional distress, relationship turmoil, physical problems (such as high blood pressure, ulcers, back pain), and global functional impairment. Like fear, however, anger can also be adaptive when it results in the identification of a problem followed by a healthy, constructive change.

In most cases, anger is a secondary emotion, which serves as the outward manifestation of a primary emotion that is under the surface (that is, not in one's consciousness). For example, when we feel scared, shamed, or wounded by another, it can be quite uncomfortable to experience the vulnerability associated with these difficult and complex feelings. Instead, the unconscious mind defensively buries these raw emotions, and anger is what rises to the top as the conscious feeling state. When working with patients, it is helpful to lead them to identifying the precursor thoughts and feelings that they were having (but often are not aware of) right before a wave of anger overcomes them. In almost all cases, patients uncover thoughts involving fear, shame, or hurt.

When it comes to raising a child, parents are certainly no strangers to the emotion of anger. You have been angry with your child for a host of reasons ranging from breaking a valuable possession and not doing his chores to lying to you and disobeying your rules. The common theme that tends to be associated with anger from a parent is the frustration and disappointment that arises when a child does something that a parent finds displeasing or unacceptable. When a parent reacts with anger to their child who is coming out to them, there are often two tacit concepts (that may not even be held consciously) intrinsically linked with the anger: (1) that their child is making a choice and (2) that there child is "doing this to them." If you are a parent who has felt anger toward your child, it is important that you take a moment to acknowledge the possibility that you are making these two assumptions. Let's take a look at each one and examine the possible reasons you may have arrived here.

First, the "choice" to be gay is actually not a choice at all. In Chapter 2, I discussed how sexuality is not something that one can choose, but rather it is due to a complex combination of variables (including one's genes, to a significant degree) that is outside of one's control. If you are still having a hard time internalizing this concept, you may have difficulty working past your anger (and guilt, for that matter). You need to fully embrace the concept that your child didn't "do this" but rather it is something for which she or he is no more responsible than athletic ability or intelligence. Just as it would be totally illogical to get angry with your child for not having curly hair, you should realize that it is equally unsound to be upset with him or her for being gay. The sooner you internalize this concept, the easier it will be to work through these stages.

Second, the idea that your child being gay is something that she or he is "doing to you" is both egocentric and flawed. By making your child's sexuality about you instead of your son or daughter, you are sending the message that your feelings are more important than your child's during this milestone life event. As a parent, I am sure you have spent most of your life putting your child's needs and feelings before yours. This situation should not be an exception. Realizing and accepting the reality that one is gay is often a difficult and elaborate process through which an individual evolves. The fear of not obtaining a parent's love and support is probably one of the biggest roadblocks that can prevent someone from working through the final steps of coming out. You may not realize this (and at times it may not seem so), but the primary goal of most children is the attainment of their parents' approval. Your child may already feel worried that you are going to be upset or disappointed when you learn that he or she is gay. If you react to your son's or daughter's coming out with anger and a statement implying that your child is somehow harming you with this news, it will be very hard to cultivate an ongoing sense of connectedness with him or her. It is imperative that you let go of the idea that your child's sexuality will adversely affect your life. In Chapter 7, I will take this concept even one step further and discuss how having a gay child will actually enhance, not detract from, the quality of your life.

Besides being angry with their child for being gay, I have worked with parents who have been angry at their child for having waited so long to come out to them. In most cases, the anger in this circumstance is one that is masking feelings of hurt and guilt for not having been there to help their child through the stages of the coming-out process. Some parents may misconstrue a child's delay in coming out to them as a lack of trust between them. These parents express anger at their child (and also at themselves) because they feel that they were left out from a significant part of their child's life. They berate themselves with the notion that they have failed in some way as a parent. My response to them is that they need to understand just how difficult it can be for a child to come out to his parent. It has been demonstrated that most children tell parents fairly late (years) into their coming-out process. Closeted gay teenagers are generally burdened by deeply entrenched self-hatred due to the secret of their sexuality. It often takes a long time to work through those feelings and rebuild their self-esteem around this newly realized facet of their identity. Furthermore, gay children feel incredibly vulnerable when coming out to their parents, and it takes time to work up the courage to do this.

Consequently, you should also cut yourself some slack if it takes you some time to fully comprehend and accept your child's homosexuality. You are just starting on a journey that they may have started on years ago, and it will take you some time to catch up. In fact, I often advise parents to tell their child something like, "I am so grateful that you feel comfortable sharing this with me. I will always love and support you, but it may take me a little while to wrap my mind around this new information because it wasn't something that I expected." You should never tell your child that you are upset with him or her for not coming out to you sooner, as it is not productive or helpful. Instead, try to understand that your child likely had reasons for waiting, and feel grateful that he ultimately did arrive at a place where he was comfortable sharing this part of himself with you.

On more than a few occasions, parents have told me that they feel anger or hostility toward some third party for either "making their child gay" or persuading her to act on homosexual impulses. In one situation, a parent blamed the faculty advisor (a gay man) of her son's Gay Straight Alliance club at school. In another, a parent insisted that her daughter's friend's older sister (a lesbian) had "led her down that pathway." The reality is, however, that no one made your child gay. It is not something that is determined by association or influence. Homosexuality is not a club that seeks new members. Rather than feeling angry with people who have likely supported your child during his coming-out process, you should sublimate that anger into gratitude for the fact that your child likely had guidance and support from others who have had similar experiences. It is often these meaningful relationships that make gay adolescents feel less alone on their journey. If your child has not been lucky enough to come into contact with gay role models, you should take the initiative of helping him or her find gay people in various phases of life who can serve as mentors. Even in big cities (like New York) with significant gay populations, it can be surprisingly difficult for closeted teenagers to find the support they need in the form of successful and well-adjusted gay adults.

I have worked with people who blamed their co-parent for having a gay child. I haven't noticed a consistent pattern in this paradigm. For example, in some cases, a mother will assert that if her husband hadn't worked so many long hours and instead spent more time playing catch in the backyard or taken him away on "boys' weekends," their son would be more masculine and attracted to women. Conversely, some fathers will allude to the fact that their overbearing wives coddled their son too much, thereby feminizing him, which resulted in him being gay. Again, and not to beat this basic but critical concept to death, no one made your child gay. A child's coming out is a major life event that has reverberations within the entire family. The degree of stress and conflict that your child perceives associated with his coming out will affect his overall perception of himself and the feelings he has about what being gay means in the context of the family unit. In short, this is a time for you and your spouse to be supporting each other's feelings and not pointing fingers or looking to place blame. Stressful events within a family generally expose vulnerabilities in relationships (that is, the prevalence of divorce following the death of a young child is quite high). If your marriage has underlying difficulties, they may come to the surface at this time. If this is the case, and you notice increased tension between you and your spouse following your child's coming out, it is crucial that you make active efforts to work on your relationship, either between the two of you or, more likely, in a therapist's office.

Many of you may be reading this book after already reacting with anger toward your child who came out to you. If that is the case, fear not, for there are still things that you can do or say to mitigate your prior actions. Here are a few simple steps you can take to improve the relationship between you and your child and ensure that your child knows that he has your love and support.

First, apologize: It is okay if your first reaction to your child's coming out was anger.

As I said before, perhaps you weren't expecting this at all and didn't have the time or the equanimity to work through your complex emotions. Once your anger has subsided, you must first apologize to your child. It always amazes me how many parents skip this step. Your child needs to know that you are sorry and that you feel bad for the hurtful things you said. A sample apology could be: "I am so incredibly sorry that I yelled at you last week when you came out to me. I deeply regret saying those things and feel horrible that I hurt you."

Second, get your lines right.

It is important that you are very mindful of the things you say to your child in the weeks and months following her coming out, as she will likely be exquisitely sensitive and looking for meaning in your word choice and tone.

If, prior to your child's coming out, for example, you had voiced some biased or prejudiced concepts about gay people, now would be the time to explain to your child that you are going to work on shifting your attitudes and biases, but that it may take some time. Make sure your child knows that you still see him the same way you did before he came out to you. Your child may feel like he is suddenly defined by his sexuality and that all of his achievements and accomplishments from the past have been erased from your memory. The core personality traits and attributes are not different at all. Remind your child of why you are proud of him or her. For example, you might say, "You are an amazing person, and I am so grateful that I have the privilege of being your mother. I have always admired your tenacious work effort at school, the loyalty you exhibit toward your friends, and incredible care and concern you have for those less fortunate than yourself. Being gay does not change any of these things."

Third, actions speak louder than words. Now is the time when you should not only be saying the right things, but take the extra step and show your child that you are invested in being the parent of a gay child.

There are many things that you can do to demonstrate your support, such as joining PFLAG, reading books on this topic, becoming politically active in gay rights issues, and marching in your city's Gay Pride parade. I understand that many parents may take years to feel comfortable enough with the situation and themselves to do some of these things, but you'll be surprised just how far a little gesture will go with your child. She will feel cared for and understood simply by seeing you reading a book such as this because it will demonstrate that you are actively making efforts to understand her better and make some changes in the way you think and act.

Anger should never be ignored or bottled up. However, it is also not reasonable to feel like you are justified in having uncontrolled, violent outbursts either. The most effective way to manage anger is to maintain a sense of control, analyze what is underlying the anger, identify the emotions and thoughts that are really at work, and then brainstorm for ways to channel the anger into something healthy or productive. As a psychiatrist, my major concern with unresolved anger is that it can some-times be turned inward and result in a depressive episode (after all, Freud defined depression as "anger turned inward"). While it is normal to feel some degree of anger for having a gay child, if, in association with intense and consuming anger, you are experiencing any of the following things, I would advise that you make an appointment for a consultation with a mental health professional because you may be experiencing a major depressive episode or a severe anxiety disorder:

- Inability to fall asleep or remain asleep for at least a week
- Loss of appetite and/or weight loss without trying to do so
- Feelings of extreme hopelessness and a sense of doom
- Inability to concentrate on work or family duties
- Feeling down or sad all the time
- No longer finding enjoyment in things or activities that you previously enjoyed
- Thoughts of wishing you were dead and/or actual ideas of wanting to harm yourself
- Feeling consumed by intense worry or concern that bad things are going to happen to you or your family.

In our next chapter, we will talk about shame, which afflicts many straight parents because of what society and their parents have taught them about homosexuality. They may feel "less than" other families and long for their old standing within the community.

· 5 ·

SHAME TO PRIDE

*"If we can share our story with someone who responds with
empathy and understanding, shame can't survive."*

—American author Brené Brown (born 1965)

SOME PARENTS FEEL shame at first after their children come out. I know I did. I wasn't *ashamed* of our son, but did feel ashamed that our family wasn't mainstream anymore. Suddenly, I had a minority child. I felt "less than" other families and longed for our old standing within our community.

I felt as if I were hiding a secret from others, lest they judge me. I eventually dropped this "soul-eating emotion" as Carl Jung defines shame, as other parents successfully have.

The following straight parents, as well as gay and lesbian children, discovered, in similar ways, how happy and relieved they and their children are to be themselves. By integrating their sexual orientation into their own lives, the family can ultimately be proud.

That being said, it may be indicative of society's prejudice and shaming that the majority of the people I interviewed wanted their name changed, whether to protect their child's privacy or their own, proving that it is still hard to be totally OUT. Also, the majority of the lesbian and gay children I interviewed first came out to their friends, and next to their mother, and they told her not to share the information with Dad. They were not only afraid of the father's wrath but also of profoundly disappointing the head of the household!

Marilyn Cusack, Daughter, Thirty-Nine

After having three sons, Marilyn's mother prayed for a little girl with flaxen hair and blue eyes. A Presbyterian Sunday School teacher originally from Ohio, her prayers were answered! What she didn't receive were the coping skills for raising a child who would later identify as a lesbian and make faces at the thought of wearing dresses—less Sara Crewe in *A Little Princess* than Scout Finch in *To Kill a Mockingbird*.

Marilyn knew she was *different* as far back as the third grade, when she had crushes on girls. However, she couldn't label that feeling until she was eighteen and realized she was a lesbian.

While in youth fellowship, she asked her leader why homosexuality was considered sinful. The teacher, who seemed uncomfortable with the question, couldn't answer Marilyn, but when Marilyn graduated from high school, the teacher gave her a book with biblical passages about homosexuality. Marilyn found the book depressing and shameful.

In high school, Marilyn dated boys, although her relationships were always platonic. At that point, she was not *out*, and because she was a jock, she was known as a tomboy. Another girl in her high school was suspected of being a lesbian, and rumors focused on that girl—not Marilyn, who was relieved although she felt a tinge of guilt for not sharing the brunt of the homophobic slurs.

Marilyn presented as a trim, attractive blonde, neither a "femme" nor a so-called lipstick lesbian, nor "butch" (masculine, usually with short hair and no makeup). She looked, and still looks, like the model in an old-fashioned soap commercial. Marilyn affirms that her looks deceive potential mates, as they initially think she's either heterosexual or bisexual, and sometimes she becomes, regrettably, "the experiment."

She attended a community college in Florida, but after a semester decided to go into the military, as her parents had done. Now, while truly living on her own, she knew that the different feeling she had had all along could be labeled: She was a lesbian. As a private in the army, she was happy, but she also feared for her safety because she might be found out. Her then-girlfriend was about to enlist. After ten months, she decided to leave, as "Don't Ask, Don't Tell" was in effect, and Marilyn knew that there was no way that she and her girlfriend could keep their love a secret. She went home.

Marilyn thought she was doomed. Her mother, as it turned out, was sympathetic about Marilyn leaving the army, until she found out the real reason for Marilyn's withdrawal. Her daughter left the army because her "friend," whom her mother knew, was more than a friend! Marilyn had come clean. It was a personal necessity, a release of an internal pressure she could no longer hide.

Like many straight parents, Marilyn's mother went into denial mode: "It's just a phase. You'll date again; you haven't found the right guy!" Marilyn, like her mother, wished it was a phase and that her orientation would go away.

But she knew it wouldn't. Marilyn was depressed not only for herself, but also for her mother. She realized she was disappointing her mother. "I had imagined my life with a man," she confided. "I felt horrible being the only girl in the family and being a lesbian. Sometimes I do feel bad and wish it were different for me and them. I see friends happily married with children, and I'm upset sometimes that I don't have the same things."

Despondent, Marilyn, was on the brink of suicide. Her life was a drama, and her phone in her room became a *deus ex machina* when it rang, distracting her as she was thinking of suicide. Marilyn took it as an omen not to self-destruct.

Marilyn moved out of her family's house in 1998. Today, she has a successful power-washing business and has a girlfriend.

How did she go from suicide ideation from feeling such shame to pride and self-confidence? "I feel much better being out and not lying to people. My sexuality does not define me."

And how is her relationship with her mother and stepfather? It took Marilyn's mother a while to accept Marilyn's orientation, but she came around, as many parents do because of their love for their child.

"My mother made it very clear that she loved me no matter what. That's what I needed to hear." Now, her mother is her best friend, to whom she can tell *anything*. Her mother is no longer ashamed, hiding her daughter's identity, nor is she confused or hoping that Marilyn will be with a man. However, she does tell her daughter jokingly to get artificially inseminated so she can have grandchildren.

According to Marilyn, "Communication is key between parent and child. You have to sit down and talk, answer the hard and uncomfortable questions, and parents have to ask them as well."

Children who throw their coming-out in their family's face and present it as a one-sided conflict often experience difficulties. Parents and siblings need the time to digest the situation. "The gay or lesbian child did not ask for this and has most likely gone through a hell of emotions to sort it all out. It's no one's fault, it's the way we are made. Parents have to realize this," Marilyn advises. However, it can take time to digest new information, and a child introducing her sexuality to family and friends can expect the best results if she approaches the topic as respectfully as possible.

Tyler Yeagley, Son, Twenty-Three

Adolescents, out of anger or despair, can blurt out they are gay in the strangest places at the most inopportune times. Not Tyler—who, at age thirteen, premeditated his unique coming-out. He decided to come out to his mother on the wedding day of her second marriage. By doing so, he thought, she wouldn't judge him; she'd be distracted and happy. Her only response? She knew he was gay. To his mother, Tyler's coming out could not have been more inconvenient.

Like Marilyn Cusack, Tyler, originally from Northern California, knew he was *different* as far back as elementary school. In high school, he entertained the idea that he could be *bisexual* as he was dating girls, and not platonically. But by age fifteen, Tyler had an epiphany: "I'm not bisexual; I'm gay!" As Tyler shared, "It was like putting glasses on. It made me sharper. I had moments of clarity."

Tyler's new X-ray vision about his orientation was not well received in his high school, located in a blue-collar town in which probably 40 percent of the families live under the poverty level. He was mercilessly harassed: On the bus, other students threw bottles of urine at him. When he tried to start a Gay-Straight Alliance at another school, he received hate mail. His mother told him to "tone it down." An altercation with a homophobic student resulted in a broken nose and Tyler's decision to leave school during his senior year.

No one had his back except his art teachers. "I was a theater nerd," confesses Tyler, who used to stay at school until 11 p.m. to avoid spending much time at his home, which had become dysfunctional. His father died when Tyler was ten. His mother was a "basket case" from the collapse of her second short-lived marriage.

To obtain a high school degree, Tyler was homeschooled. Although he received extra attention from his mother for lessons, she struggled to maintain discipline, feeling sidetracked by her own problems. Tyler was allowed to smoke and drink when he was fifteen, and he brought home boyfriends. His mother, feeling out of control and fed up with his lifestyle, kicked him out of the house. Tyler said she left "just when I needed her most. I needed a shoulder to lean on, support and sympathy." His emotions were bruised, perhaps permanently.

It was the pain of nonrecognition. Although his mother has since apologized for his expulsion, and he has forgiven her, she has nevertheless papered over the problems associated with embarrassment and hurt.

When they do talk, it is angry and one-sided, with their voices scraping and grinding against each other. The bitterness of unresolved issues is still evident in their communications. "Our relationship is rocky," states Tyler. The largest issue he has with his mother is that "she believes it's okay to be gay but not to talk about it to others. She's only supportive when we're alone."

Tyler feels he should get equal airtime with his brother, eleven years older, and his sister, seven years younger. He feels he shouldn't have to jostle for his mother's attention, and that the issues he has that are related to sexuality shouldn't be invalidated just because his mother doesn't want to discuss them. "The more she and others talk about having a gay family member, the more normal it becomes."

In the past, Tyler has brought a boyfriend to family meals at which the lover is introduced as Tyler's "friend." Everyone dances around the issue of his being gay. He has given up including his boyfriends in family celebrations and wonders who will show up to his wedding on July 31, 2016.

Tyler believes that if his mother had talked to someone who has a gay son, she would have been better off. He wishes that his mother could have maintained a parental role, guiding and supporting him through life. "Instead," he said, "she turned me into her therapist. I felt like a pseudo *spouse*."

According to Tyler, parents shouldn't blame their son or daughter. It's nobody's fault that the child is gay. The parent shouldn't feel shame, nor should the child. "You're not being punished," points out Tyler. "He or she is the same child that you've always loved. Gay should not be regarded as bad or imperfect, nor should it be a disappointment."

"My shame," says Tyler," has put armor around my heart. "I've had to peel back that armor." As Tyler explains, guilt can be healthy, as it can make you consider a change in your life. However, shame just makes you feel bad and unworthy.

From the ages of sixteen to nineteen, Tyler learned how to penetrate that protective armor in shame workshops at Empty Closets, Inc., an online community of resources and a safe place to chat for LGBT persons. Tyler did peer counseling at the organization and eventually became a board member. In therapy, he also studied the shame-resilience research of best-selling authors Pia Mellody and Brené Brown and has listened to a variety of helpful TED talks online.

Today, Tyler is planning on obtaining an masters in social work and is part-owner of a health and wellness practice in Sacramento, Inner Harmony Healing, where he is a life coach, focusing on dealing with shame and vulnerability. A licensed masseur, he does somato-emotional therapy, which releases from the body the held-in energy of trauma through mind and bodywork.

Jacob Thomas, Son, Twenty-Five

You don't want to be gay, raised in the Pentecostal Church, and be from northern Georgia. Jacob Thomas, who now lives in Minneapolis, knows the pitfalls only too well. Like Marilyn and Tyler, he felt *different* at age seven or eight.

When he understood, between the ages of ten and twelve, that his same-sex attraction was never going to disappear, he cried himself to sleep at night and prayed that this "evil, sick, shameful" lust that he hated would magically leave him. Jesus wasn't helping him.

It has taken him twenty-two years to come to terms with his sexuality and to realize that he can't change it. It is who he is, he didn't choose it, and he can't fight it. There is no point in denying it, but for a long time he did just that.

When Jacob was fifteen, a boy he knew in another school sent him a letter that Jacob's mother found and interpreted as a love letter. (Jacob had been corresponding with this boy, but that boy's parents never found Jacob's letters.) Although Jacob and this adolescent later identified as gay, they didn't know they were gay at the time.

Still in denial, Jacob's mother dragged Jacob to his Pentecostal school to meet with the school principal, who queried Jacob about the contents of the letter. Jacob told the principal, and later his church, that he was not gay, but that his friend might be, and that he and the religious leaders could *save* his friend. "I pretended that I was totally uncomfortable and was worried about his salvation." In another meeting with both sets of parents, "I totally threw him under the bus," said Jacob.

Subsequently, Jacob totally immersed himself in church so God would come save him and finally remove those feelings that he couldn't change.

Trying to settle his nagging same-sex attraction, Jacob chose the most masculine career he could think of to prove to himself that he was straight: the United States Air Force. His father, who worked for a carpet company, was delighted, as he had thought of being a history teacher and was always interested in the military. Jacob and his father used to bond by watching old war movies as well as the History Channel together.

Jacob received an associate degree in Electronics from the Community College of the U.S. Air Force in Grand Forks, North Dakota. During that time, he was a computer network technician in the air force. He also volunteered at a local church as a sound technician. He is now in the air force reserves as of May 2014, having served six years in active duty. Like Marilyn, he too served during "Don't Ask, Don't Tell."

Still convinced he could be straight, Jason married in 2009 but was subsequently divorced after two years; although he didn't attribute the failure to his being gay. After divorcing, he started living as a gay man in March of 2012. "I figured I was going to hell anyway."

After his service with the Air Force, Jacob moved to gay-friendly Minneapolis, where he delved into progressive politics: working for Obama, for gay marriage in Minnesota, and for Sharon Sund's election to Congress.

For the past five years, he has been working on branding and digital strategy for small businesses and attending the University of Minnesota at which he has created his own major, Social Justice Theatre.

On June 25, 2012, Jacob formally came out in a six-minute video that you can see on RUComingOut.com. With his parents 3,000 miles away, he wanted to come out before they found out from an impersonal source such as Facebook. Jacob wanted to tell his parents first and had a phone nearby so they could talk to him about the contents of the video after they viewed it.

With the video, he couldn't be interrupted with questions from his parents. Although his parents said they would always love Jacob, they couldn't eschew their religious dogma and the belief that unless Jacob changed his ways (since they believed it was a lifestyle) he was going to end up in hell.

His parents were upset that Jacob was so public with his message, but as Jason said, "they were annoyed they didn't have more time to cover up." His mother felt betrayed. She would have preferred a private letter. His folks were asked by a Georgia friend who saw the post on Facebook, "How long have you known?"

Jacob's thirteen-year-old adopted brothers don't know he is gay. They have asked Jacob why he wears makeup when he goes out. "I have an uneasy truce with my folks. I won't lie. Should my brothers ask if I have a girlfriend, I will say 'No, I have a boyfriend.' If I'm dating a boy, don't call him a 'friend'; he's a boyfriend." Jacob is not welcome to bring a boy to his parent's house anyway.

This familial estrangement has been trying. Says Jacob, "A parent shouldn't tell you how you feel and try to convince you that you are straight." Jacob's mother told him, "When you were thirteen, you had a crush on Meagan." Or, "You can't be gay. You were married and told us at age fifteen that you weren't gay."

The nasty cocktail of guilt, embarrassment, and hurt on his parents' part shouldn't, in Jacob's eyes, prevent them from asking Jacob about his boyfriend. "Even if they regard homosexuality as a sin, they can still love the sinner and show interest in my significant other, as it's important to me." It's hurtful not to acknowledge someone who's important to you. They are not betraying their religion if your parents say, "We like your partner," or give your boyfriend a hug.

It's okay for parents to say, "I need to process this information and will work hard to have a healthy relationship with you." As Jacob put it, "My mother said she would not have sent me to a straight camp, that's a conversion camp, but I knew she would have sent me to a religious therapist who would have tried to convert me to straight, so what's the difference?"

Jacob adds that "gay and lesbian children should not only get the message that they are loved but also that they are not damaged or 'less than.' Plenty of gay people have become successful." He says, "It's important to get yourself out of your mindset so you can really listen to your child. You can do this by going to an affirming LGBT therapist, reading books, educating yourself online, for example. Ask yourself, what would it look like if you did affirm?"

Stephanie Segura, Daughter, Forty

Stephanie was not out until she was twenty-four. It was no surprise to her large family, especially her mother and second oldest sister, who called her a "lesbian" whenever they would fight, although they used the term solely as an insult. And yet her sister Laurie said, after Stephanie came out, "Why didn't you tell us before?"

There's good reason why Stephanie didn't want to come out to her Roman Catholic family, and homophobic slurs were merely the icing on the cake. She felt that her family's casual use of bigoted language indicated a deeper antipathy toward homosexuals. Her father would call an actor on television a a "queer." And though both parents are civil to her gay uncle, Stephanie was frightened of her parents' reaction.

Stephanie met her wife, Becca Sicairos, at her job at gay-friendly members-only warehouse where she worked as a floor supervisor in Salt Lake City, Utah. In the beginning, she and Becca hung out but could not bring themselves to talk about their strong mutual attractions. When Stephanie's same-sex relationship broke up, she leaned on Becca for support, even though she knew Becca dated men. They became close.

After two years, Becca and Stephanie were unprepared to

address their same-sex attraction. Stephanie texted Becca, "I am having feelings I probably should not have for you." She felt shame. She did not want to lose her closest pal and thought she may have been overly flirtatious. But in time, Becca and Stephanie realized that they were both interested in each other and began seeing each other romantically. They kept their relationship secret at work because Becca's mother also worked at the warehouse, and they felt she would not approve. Becca and Stephanie proceeded slowly.

There were complications. Stephanie grew up a tomboy and knew before she was thirteen that she was attracted to girls. Becca had never been in a relationship with a woman. She worried about how her tight-knit family would react.

Not only did their friendship survive; it blossomed. "The seriousness of their relationship pointed to a desire to have a family and not just be a couple." They had two children: Ellie, one, and Brayden, now three.

On December 27, 2014, they married in Utah. They were able to squeak in after December 20, when a federal district court judge found Utah's voter-approved ban on same-sex marriages unconstitutional and barred the state from blocking them. Later, Utah became the eighteenth state, along with the District of Columbia, to allow same-sex marriage.

Like many parents, Stephanie's don't like to talk about issues affecting LGBT people. Her mother changes the subject when it's brought up. "They don't support me," says Stephanie, who cries about the situation to her oldest sister, who is more sympathetic. "Nothing has changed."

"Parents should stand up for their gay kids. If my parents' priest tells the congregation that it's wrong for same-sex couples to marry, then my folks should confront him and find another parish. My folks should listen to the gay child and love people who they are." Like Meagan O'Nan (see page 63), Stephanie's mother was embarrassed to introduce Becca as Stephanie's wife. It made me feel awful. "We consider ourselves married, and we have two kids, and they can't take that away from us."

Dorothy Russell, Mother, Sixty

"I'm ashamed of what I did years ago," confessed Dorothy Russell. "At age ten, I thought Kevin was effeminate. He wasn't like other boys; he lisped. His gait was different; I suspected that he was gay, so I tried to change him. I hung Cindy Crawford posters in his room to try to redirect him."

Dorothy didn't know better. Even though she lives near San Francisco "in a town known for its hippies, liberals and farmers," she herself was not accepting of Kevin's sexual orientation. With no role models or gay family members in her own adoptive family, she needed a blueprint for understanding.

When she confronted Kevin about the gay websites she found on the computer, he said, "I bookmarked them so you'd know I was gay." Although Dorothy had a sneaking suspicion that her son was gay, the confirmation was too much for her to bear. It shook up her expectations. She woke her husband, Roger, and told him, "Kevin is gay." He wasn't as nonplussed and retorted, "So, Kevin is gay."

She obviously took the news much harder than her husband, an environmental health chief, who was more concerned about Kevin's safety than anything else. For that reason, Dorothy told Kevin to stay in the closet his sophomore year due to the harassment he might receive in sports. Roger did keep it a secret at his job and was not pleased when he heard from a friend that he "saw your son dressed as a girl at Denny's."

As many parents do once their child comes out, they retreated into the closet. Daughter Madison was away at college when Kevin came out. When he came out to his friends and family members, Dorothy told Kevin that he had to tell his sister, but she didn't want Madison to discuss Kevin's same-sex orientation with friends.

Kevin was questioning his sexuality as early as junior high school. He had few friends and seemed depressed. His counselor didn't deal with sexual orientation, and during junior high, Dorothy was frightened that Kevin might commit suicide.

He did, however, have a girlfriend in ninth grade, which gave his mother hope for a so-called *normal* life. "I asked him if he had any sexual experiences, and Kevin said no." But when he came out, her dreams of having grandchildren and seeing her son get married were withered. "I couldn't see beyond those expectations. That took a long time to lose."

"I must have cried for nine months—in the bathroom at my dentist's office and in the car." Dorothy felt as if she were on a hamster wheel going nowhere.

Unfortunately, Kevin saw her tears, and she realized that it wasn't fair to him. She made herself a promise to appear as a well-adjusted parent of a gay son. "He shouldn't have been made to feel ashamed that he had caused my disappointment."

While Dorothy was crying, Kevin was blossoming. He attended a Positive Images Group, a therapy-oriented group that also included transgendered young people and proved to be helpful for adolescents.

Free to be himself after being out, Kevin became popular. He started a Gay-Straight Alliance at his high school, won a volunteer award, and had the self-confidence to take a boy to the prom without notifying the school first. After high school, Kevin received a BA from University of California, Santa Cruz, and is now a successful accountant.

Dorothy, concerned about her standing within the community as the mother of a gay son, decided to go a therapist who happened to be a lesbian. The mental health worker gave her books about raising gay children and suggested she attend PFLAG meetings. Gradually, Dorothy learned to let go of her outmoded expectations for Kevin and learned to accept him as he is. She is President of a PFLAG chapter in Santa Rosa, California.

Once ashamed of having a gay son, now Dorothy refers gay people in the community to her dental office, where she is a dental hygienist. Now the dentist office is known as the office for the gay community because of her enthusiastic support. She can't stop talking about how proud she is of her gay son.

Parents, recommends Dorothy, should educate themselves first, digest the material, then go back and say to their gay child, "I totally understand. You should remember that you are the parent, and don't let your child see you crying. He has enough weight of his burden."

THE DOCTOR IS IN

Are you experiencing shame? If you agree with any of these statements, then you are probably struggling with shame:

1. Personally, I am comfortable with the fact that my daughter is a lesbian, but I don't feel the need to tell the neighbors.
2. I completely support gay marriage, but I still wish my son were straight.
3. I am thrilled that my son is married to his partner, but I could never introduce him as his "husband."
4. I just want to make sure that the church doesn't find out that Raymond is gay because I am not sure they will allow me to continue to attend.

Like guilt, shame is a negative emotion that arises when we feel bad about some aspect of our lives, our actions, or ourselves. However, in the case of guilt, we feel badly because we have not lived up to our *own* standards or values, whereas with shame, we feel that we have not met *societal* or *cultural* expectations. Shame arises when we feel that our personal defects or flaws are exposed to the community at large. Another differentiation is that guilt tends to be limited to an action that we have taken or not taken, whereas shame is a pervasive negative emotion about how we feel overall. It is quite common for parents of gay children to feel ashamed at some point simply for having a child who is gay. This stems from the fact that on some level many people feel that being gay is unnatural and/or outside the norms of society.

There are two operating assumptions when a parent feels ashamed for having a gay child. First is the notion that your child is an extension of yourself and that people will judge you for qualities in your child. It is important to realize that you and your child are separate entities and that it is neither right nor fair for you to view your child as a part of yourself. Doing so puts tremendous pressure on him to meet your expectations for what you think he should be. It also makes it more likely that you will expend energy worrying about what people think of your child, and fear that they may think poorly of you. I have worked with countless parents who have come to me in great distress over how some third party (for example, family, friends, and church members) will view their child. I have found that in these situations, the parents are actually more concerned about what these people will think of *them*, not their child, and some self-reflection will reveal underlying insecurities that they need to overcome.

The second assumption parents make when they feel ashamed for having a gay child is that being gay is somehow inferior or undesirable. Shame is only experienced in situations where one feels that some quality of theirs is universally viewed by others as worthy of embarrassment. Understanding how and why you have come to view being gay as shameful is something that you will need to spend some time on, either through self-reflection or work with a therapist. There are often underlying biases or personal experiences that contribute to the shame parents may experience in having a gay child. For example, I worked with a man who had been bullied as a child because he wasn't good at sports. Peers would mock him for "throwing like a girl," and he was generally ostracized for lacking traditional masculine qualities. To overcome his resultant low self-esteem, he took up bodybuilding in college and spent a tremendous amount of time and energy getting into excellent shape. Although he was no longer teased (and, in fact, often received adulation for his physique), he was unable to work past the childhood taunts and still viewed himself as being weak and unmasculine. Having a gay son activated his shame button because he feared that people would mock his son for being gay, which would, in turn, reflect on him. Once he was able to separate these two distinct experiences in his mind, he was able to work past his shame and come to the realization that having a gay son in no way detracted from his own masculinity.

In my experience working with parents, I have found that shame is more often latent, particularly in the case of parents who are the most overtly accepting of having a gay child. In this situation, shame is generally not conscious but is evident in their actions. For example, I worked with one family in which the mother never expressed an iota of protest or distress upon learning that her son was gay. A few years later, however, when it came to introducing her son's husband to friends or strangers, she had an extremely difficult time uttering the word "husband." She would either avoid it, simply stating, "This is

Tom," or "Meet my son-in-law." When her son pointed out this pattern of avoidance, she felt terrible and was disappointed in herself, but she couldn't come up with a satisfactory explanation for why it made her uncomfortable. She said that she was worried that it would make the other person feel awkward, so in order to spare that person any discomfort, she avoided using the word. Ultimately, she realized that it was her own discomfort, which she was projecting onto others, that was causing her to behave this way. Upon deeper exploration, she uncovered the feeling of shame as the root of her discomfort.

I have also encountered the paradoxical scenario of liberal parents who are fully supportive of gay rights and gay marriage, and may even have close gay friends, but are not accepting of their own gay child. These patients express an irrational desire for their child to be straight. In this situation, parents connect intellectually with the concept of equal rights for everyone and recognize that gay people are no different from straight people and thus should be treated equitably in our society. Despite their egalitarian beliefs, however, they continue to harbor an emotional preference toward having straight children of their own. In some ways, these parents actually struggle more than conservative parents because they have the extra burden of needing to reconcile contradictory beliefs, which contributes to added emotional distress and cognitive dissonance. It is especially difficult for these parents because, first, they need to bring to consciousness their latent shame for having a gay child and, then, they need to work on forgiving themselves for feeling that way.

Tacit shame can manifest as a lack of engagement with your child about his sexuality when he comes out to you. For example, when your child tells you he is gay, you should be sure to check in with him regularly about how the coming-out process is going. I referred in the previous chapter to the concept of needing to "get your lines right," and by that I mean saying the right thing to your child immediately after his coming out to you. However, many parents incorrectly think it ends there, and, that as long as they have done that, they have completed their duty as a parent of a gay child. The reality is that the next step—the follow-through—is just as important as the first. Here are some examples of questions or conversation starters you can use with your child to demonstrate that you are interested in this aspect of his life and are not ashamed of having a gay child.

"How do you feel about being gay?"

Many gay people themselves need to work through their own shame about being gay before they can start the process of coming out to others. Moreover, for some, managing the shame can be an ongoing lifelong process. The best way for you to help your child work through her own shame is by making it clear that you yourself are not ashamed. I have found that shame tends to be contagious. There are ways in which you may be perpetuating your child's shame without even realizing it. One parent became angry with his child who was being teased at school for the way he dressed and the interests he expressed. Instead of defending his child, the parent said that his son shouldn't wear "girly" colors and should make more of an effort to pretend to like sports so the boys wouldn't bully him. Although the parent had the best intention and was only trying to minimize the teasing and distress, he sent a message that reinforced his child's shame by not encouraging his son to be himself. Your children—both gay and straight—need to know that you are unambiguously on their side and willing to protect them.

"Who have you told so far that you are gay, and how have they reacted?"

It is rather likely that you are not the first person in whom your child confided about his sexuality, so you should make an effort to get brought up to speed. There is no better way than showing your child you are engaged in their coming-out process than by asking about how people have reacted and what impact it has had on those relationships. One of the hardest aspects of coming out is the fear that lifelong relationships are going to suddenly shift or shatter upon sharing your news. Your child will feel understood and supported if you convey your understanding of this difficult process and will appreciate your support as a parent.

"How has being gay affected your life, and has it changed your vision of your future?"

I spoke in previous chapters about not making assumptions regarding how your child's life will unfold simply because she is gay. A neutral, nonjudgmental way to initiate this conversation is to say something such as, "It's so great that, in this day and age, gay people can have all of the things in their lives that straight people can have, especially now that gay marriage is legal and more and more gay people are starting families of their own. Have you given any thought to what you want for yourself? We will support you in any way we can to help you accomplish whatever your heart desires." This is a nice way to make your child feel supported and unjudged and to get to know what your child wishes for her own life. Also, keep in mind that it is highly likely that your child's concept of his future may change as he or she matures. Many straight teenage boys say that they absolutely do not plan to have children but then later in life do have children because their vision of what they want for themselves evolves.

"Who haven't you told yet, and what is your plan?"

Your child may want to discuss strategies for coming out to other friends and family members. It can be particularly hard to share the news with older family members from a different era. You may say something like, "Have you thought about telling Grandma? If you'd like me to help you figure out how to do that or to be there when you tell her, just let me know. I would love to help make that easier." I will discuss this in more detail in the Chapter 7 (see page 187).

Many parents think they just need to ask the requisite questions as if they are checking off a list; then they become complacent and feel they have done all they need to do. However, you have to remember that coming out is a process, not a procedure. You may ask your child if she wants to talk about something on one day, and she may say no; then on another day, she may subtly bring something up and wait for you to ask her questions. It is best to ask open-ended questions that encourage longer, more substantive responses. It is also important to accept the possibility that even if you provide a totally open and receptive forum for conversation, your child may still not want to talk to you about this topic for a while. Some straight teenagers refuse to talk to their parents about sex, dating, or relationships because they just don't feel comfortable doing so. This is not necessarily pathologic, so you shouldn't personalize it, get angry, or feel rejected. Always be sure to keep the door open, because you never know when your child may choose to walk through it. I once worked with a father who tried to be extremely supportive of his son during the months following his child's coming out, but the son rebuffed his parent's efforts, either answering the father's questions with a single word or just walking out of the room. The father personalized the rejection and decided he never again would ask questions pertaining to his son's sexuality. About a year later, the son began to subtly re-engage with his father, but because the father was still shut down, he did not pick up on his son's cues, and his son ultimately felt rejected and then he disengaged again. My advice to parents, therefore, is never to shut the door to the possibility of connecting with your child because it will most likely happen on his or her terms, not yours.

Some parents with whom I have worked have been concerned about how friends and colleagues will react to their having a gay child. They feel that they will be judged or possibly rejected, so they may avoid the topic or actively try to keep it a secret as if it is something for which to be ashamed. If you are worried about how others will treat you because you have a gay child, you need to reexamine the nature and strength of your relationships in the same way you would tell your child to do if one of her friends suddenly rejected her upon finding out she was gay. Just as your child should, you, too, should tell people proudly. If you think you are going to have a hard time accomplishing this, you should practice what you are going to say. I worked with a parent who is an actor, and she used to practice what she was going to say to people in front of a mirror just as she rehearsed lines for a play. I have found that most people will react in a way that parallels the manner in which you share the news. If you seem uncomfortable and ashamed, then they will react awkwardly; but if you share the news with pride and comfort, they will genuinely feel happy for you. Even if you seem comfortable, some people may have negative reactions or make insensitive remarks. However, it is important for you to maintain a healthy perspective on what matters most in your life and not to surround yourself with people who propagate shameful feelings.

· 6 ·

LOSS TO GAIN

"Life can only be understood backwards,
but it must be lived forwards."

—Danish philosopher Søren Kierkegaard (1813–1855)

WITH THE EXCEPTION of Katy Bourne, mentioned in Chapter 4, all parents I interviewed experienced a deep sadness once they found out a child was gay, almost a mourning over what feels like the loss of an "ideal" child. I know I experienced loss myself and recognize that it is a valid emotion.

When you're a new parent, you may not envision the possibility that your child could be gay. Consequently, a parent builds a lifetime of dreams and expectations for that child that often include marrying the opposite sex and having biological children. When these dreams, built on years of hopes, are dashed by a child's coming-out, a profound disappointment occurs. Of course, parents still love their child, but must—as I learned also—alter and reevaluate their expectations for their gay/lesbian kids so they can forge new relationships based not only on honesty, but also on reality. Once these expectations are adjusted, parents will be able to perceive a brighter future for their children.

Similarly, LGBT children feel a sense of loss. They know

their lives will be harder. They cannot take for granted that they will be accepted everywhere. Many are reluctant to come out to their parents, as they know what doing so would mean to their parents; they would be disappointing their parents' dreams for their sons and daughters that they have held since their children were infants. It's a loss for both that needs to be acknowledged and resolved so they both can progress to greater understanding.

One such gay son who was frightened to divulge his sexual identity is Richard Ogawa.

Richard Ogawa, Son, Thirty-Four

Officially, Richard Ogawa, originally from Seattle, then Vancouver, came out at age seventeen to his best friend, a supportive girl, in high school. He next told his sister Caroline, three years younger than he, who was "fine" with his revelation. Richard suspected in elementary school that he was gay, but by middle school, he had crushes on girls. In eighth grade, he was frequently asked, "Why do you have to act so gay?" Miserable, he began to feign sickness so he wouldn't have to go to school and be bullied. One bully reacted with disgust when Richard wore the same shirt he was wearing, shoving Richard in the hall. Richard solved the problem by giving the shirt to his sister.

"They had not invented *Will and Grace* yet; that really was the turning point in acceptance of gays," attests Richard. By high school, Richard switched from playing piano, which he started at age nine, to playing clarinet in the high school band. The band teacher "had his back" and would stop any bullying that occurred. "Theater and music gave me self-confidence," confirms Richard. Named class valedictorian, Richard had not sorted out his sexual feelings and was not in a sexual relationship with anyone.

Starting out as a day student at college in Vancouver, Richard transferred after a year to a dramatic academy in New York City. In Manhattan, he acted off-Broadway and gained the confidence to figure out his sexual orientation.

He gradually told his acting friends that he was gay, but he was afraid to disappoint his traditional Japanese parents, who were dependent on their children to translate English when they, for example, went to the bank. Richard forced himself to write a coming-out letter to his parents when he was nineteen. Nervous, he waited for his mother to respond by letter. The seventeen days it took the letter to reach him seemed interminable. Richard's mother was confused, upset, and fearful of "his choice." A month later, he went home and had a heart-to-heart talk with his mother while gardening. Long discussions followed.

As Richard pointed out to his parents, his only real choice was whether to hide his orientation or be open and ultimately be happy. He chose the latter, because he knew that if *he* were happy, they would be happy. This strategy paid off. Richard feels blessed to have parents who always had his best interest at heart and who had the courage to open their minds to non-traditional relationships, foreign to their upbringings.

Says Richard, "Perhaps if every parent toyed with the possibility that any of their children could be gay, it would change the way they raise children, period. I think the first step in parenting healthy gay children is to understand that gay children are no different; so little of their sexual orientation has to do with who they are as a whole. And I think children should be taught tolerance and acceptance and be given the freedom and the guidance to be themselves."

Since then, Richard's parents have welcomed Richard's partner, Daniel, into their home. Richard and Daniel live together in Los Angeles, where Richard works for an online streaming video website. In fact, Daniel, a banker, was one of the pallbearers at Richard father's funeral.

Cecily Condon, Mother, Seventy-Five

There is no expiration date for loss, as Cecily Condon from Raleigh, North Carolina, found out. She guesses she felt loss for five years after she found out her son Joseph was gay. Joseph, whom his mother calls "brilliant and handsome," is a successful partner at a white-shoe law firm and is married to his husband, whom he has been with for ten years. But, fearful of a possible negative reaction, Joseph did not come out until he was thirty.

Apparently, "Joey" knew he was gay when he was thirteen but denied it for a long time, immersing himself in school, both as a National Honor Society student, a Dean's List scholar at the University of North Carolina, and later as a Columbia Law student. He hoped his sexuality was a phase out of which he would grow. He shut down those yearnings while he was at college.

Cecily, who worked in human resources for a well-known company, and her husband, Frank, a former naval officer, suspected that Joey was gay, as he never wanted to meet girls at the beach. Joey also never had a girlfriend in high school, although he dated some girls. He was teased in the eighth grade and called names. To his mother and father, he also seemed depressed.

Joey came out to his parents in a long letter that stated that he had been trying to tell his folks for a long time. Cecily was visiting her sister, who had cancer, in Maryland. Frank opened the letter and read the contents to his wife over the telephone.

Immediately, Cecily instructed Frank to call Joey and tell him that they loved and accepted him. Joey, relieved, told them he thought they would be accepting, but so many of his friends *thought* their parents would be accepting, and they ended up by being rejected.

Acceptance was not a problem for Cecily and Frank, but loss was. They felt disappointment that their son wouldn't know the joy of parenting, although he and his husband, Martin, have thought of adopting a child. In particular, Cecily loves babies and children and felt sadness that she wouldn't know the fulfillment of grandparenting even though her other, younger son, Douglas, lives in Raleigh and has two children, ages twelve and fifteen.

Joseph made it clear that if anything should happen to his brother and sister-in-law, he would want to raise their children. This generous and loving attitude toward his brother's children made Cecily and Frank happy.

Cecily realized on her own timetable that she did not cause her child to be gay, nor did he choose to be gay. The Condons, who had gay friends, explained to Joey at age ten or eleven what homosexuality meant. With these epiphanies in place, the loss Cecily experienced felt like an afterthought.

Natalie, Mother, Sixty-Three

Loss can be a struggle for any parent with a gay kid, but multiply it times two, and you have a recipe for more stress. Natalie, a former Californian now living on Long Island, New York, with her ex-manufacturing husband, Arnie, discovered they had not one but two gay sons. Though the boys came out at different times, the effect of hearing that multiple offspring were gay left Natalie reeling.

"My first reaction was hurt and disbelief. I thought it must be a mistake and that my child was just confused. I also was getting mixed messages, as my eldest had a heterosexual experience at age twenty-one. Frankly, I muddled through—and not very successfully. It took a big toll on me emotionally.

It changed our life greatly. I lost weight and felt drained all the time."

The oldest son came out first. Brad, a cheerleader at a competitive boarding school, became depressed and anxious before coming out to his parents. He spent time curled up in the fetal position in the school infirmary. One year, on the night before he left for spring vacation, he "dropped the bomb," as he called it. His parents asked, "Are you sure?" He answered, "No, I'm not sure," and admitted that in his freshman year, he had a girlfriend.

Natalie, wondering if being gay was a choice, was upset that the family name would be a dead-end. (The family did have one additional child, a daughter—she was the first to know that her oldest brother was gay.) Natalie felt that it was a loss to the genetic pool. Arnie was more accepting and believed his son's confession to be genuine; Arnie didn't believe it was a situation that was going to change over time. Natalie, though, was still distraught. Arnie called a doctor friend, a surgeon he knew in the army, who suggested "crisis management." The doctor felt certain that their son was gay.

Their younger son, Dean, six years his brother's junior, went to a different boarding school. Dean was into drama and singing and had an active social life. He never actually came out, but his understanding of his own sexuality evolved in high school at about age fourteen, at approximately the same time as his older brother, although he was six years younger. As Natalie says, "He's not playing rugby, but is drop-dead gorgeous." Still, Dean encountered harassment in the locker room and also became depressed at school. His mother was worried he was going to hurt himself. Overshadowed by his older brother and sister, Dean was a different learner in school, says Natalie, and these issues, compounded by his unspoken turmoil over his sexuality, led him to turn to drugs and alcohol to allay his depression. Many studies have demonstrated the increased risk of drug and alcohol abuse (20 percent to 30 percent of the population) in gay and lesbian adolescents as compared to their heterosexual counterparts (9 percent of the population).

To assuage her loss, Natalie delved into private therapy. She also spoke daily to two people she was close to: her sister, and the godmother of her youngest son. Natalie had to wrestle with her Catholic religion. Her Catholic church believes it's fine to be gay as long as you don't act on it. Dean said his brother was gay in CCD class (classes provided by the Confraternity of Christian Doctrine association for the education of children in the Roman Catholic Church) and was told that he was going to hell, at which point Brad called the monsignor to complain. Natalie, whose faith is strong, now has two children who are agnostic. She continues to practice her religion and believes God loves everyone, including gays.

Natalie estimates that it took her about two years after Dean's coming out to get over the loss. Now friends, who discover that they have gay children, are coming to her for advice. Although her oldest son, now in a same-sex marriage with two children by surrogacy, would like her to march and be a PFLAG-carrying card member, she'd rather demonstrate her support quietly.

Her younger son, clean and sober, is in a relationship, and his partner is included in their annual Christmas card. Natalie and Arnie see Brad and Dean, who are in Brooklyn and Manhattan, constantly.

Alicia, Daughter, Thirty-One

"Life is too short to care about what others think, even if it's your parents," so says Alicia Sanchez, a lesbian who lives in Miami, Florida. Owner of a Kids Fashion Design and Sewing school, Alicia also designs for a women's resort-wear line.

She is the daughter of parents from the Dominican Republic, which she states made her different from most Hispanics in Florida. Dominicans are very traditional and honor a male-dominated society. Alicia lived in the Dominican Republic among her relatives while in her twenties.

Alicia was taught to make her parents proud. The only girl in her family, with two younger brothers and one older, she was pushed in both parochial and public high school to do well academically but also to be on the lookout for a husband.

In high school, she knew she was a lesbian. She would comment to her father, for example, that she didn't like a boy her father was eyeing for her, as he was not her "cup of tea." Alicia always provided excuses, as she felt that her parents would not be proud of her if she were gay. Her dad would always say, "Learn to cook this dish for your husband." He hadn't a clue about her sexual orientation.

Alicia developed cancer in college and, because of her sexual orientation, kept her distance from the parents, with whom she was once close. She kept postponing her coming out, as she knew it would be a loss for her parents and therefore a disappointment or letdown for her.

As part of her cancer treatment, she was given a psychologist as an integral part of a get-well team. Because she was anxious about coming out, she asked the psychologist how to approach her parents. Timing is everything. The psychologist advised her to ask her parents questions: *Do you think I am a good person? You have accepted me as sick? Does God accept me? Do I have a good heart?* Then came the climax: *I want to spend the rest of my life with women. I'm a lesbian.* When Alicia told her parents the news, her mother cried; her father was speechless but later hugged her. "My father's affection made that one of the best days of my life," said Alicia. "I told my parents I'd always love them." Alicia gave her mother the book *Love, Ellen*, because her mother likes Ellen DeGeneres as a television host. She hoped it would help her mother become more comfortable with lesbians in general.

Her two younger brothers were open and supportive, but her older brother, thirty-nine, who studied for the seminary and is traditional, asked her, "Why are you hurting our parents?" Alicia is careful who she brings home to Mom, fifty-five, and Poppy, fifty-six, and has no public displays of affection in front of them.

Ultimately, her parents have accepted her sexual orientation. As Alicia says, "It doesn't change who you are or make you less-than." She knew she was accepted when her father joked lightheartedly that he guessed "you won't be making this dish for your husband."

Judy Apelbaum, Mother, Fifty-Six

Judy Apelbaum, parent of Ryan Apelbaum, now a twenty-four year-old nurse, was not prepared for her son's coming out at age fourteen. She was shocked at her son's announcement.

It changed the family structure: "No white-gown wedding, no grandchild," stressed Judy. Her aspirations and expectations and years of investment in those dreams just went down the drain. "I understood that this was a lifetime loss," said Judy. "It took me a year to get over the news."

Why was she so rattled? After all, her parents were sophisticated. Her father was a dentist, a liberal Jew in the New York City area. "But it was like: not in my backyard!"

To resolve these uneasy feelings, Judy attended PFLAG meetings in New Jersey for a short time. Her husband, Murray, sixty-five and an accountant, took longer to "come around." He was told second. "Don't tell Dad yet . . ." became the family's modus operandi.

As Judy said, "People who have a tough time adjusting to their children's coming out don't know their kids well. Ryan was different from other boys in New Jersey. Even as a five-year-old, he had a sense of style and was more emotional.

He wanted to do ballet; his father wanted him to play baseball. . . . What was my problem? Why was I looking at this as a loss? The gay child is not going to get over the notion that he's gay. There doesn't have to be one way that families have to look. You don't have to have a heteronormative perspective. There are many flavors of ice creams. Every house doesn't have to have the idyllic white picket fence."

Like many parents, Judy realized that unless you want to create a long-term problem, you have to adjust. Loving your child is more important than your ego. It's not about you. She contends that if you love your child, you don't have to choose between what makes them happy and what makes you happy.

"Ryan seems happy. It's a matter of heart, not sheets. When Ryan was nineteen or twenty, he was in a gay relationship that lasted three years. The relationship would have been the same for a girl. The boyfriend embodied all I wanted for Ryan: kind, smart, loving."

Julia Welch, Daughter, Thirteen

There are exceptions—like Julia's mother, Duana C. Welch, PhD, psychology professor at a community college in Austin, Texas, and author of *Love Factually: 10 Proven Steps from I Wish to I Do*. She did not feel a deep sense of loss after discovering her daughter Julia was gay. In fact, Duana helped her own brother, now forty-five, come out. Commented Dr. Welch, who has written a blog about all kinds of relationships since 2009, "in a way, I was relieved that Julia identifies as a lesbian. I don't have to worry about Julia getting pregnant, and I'd be happy to have a daughter-in-law rather than a son-in-law."

However, Duana was surprised, because Julia was, as she described, "a girly-girl" three years ago. Now she wears all black. At age twelve, Julia came out to her mother as a bisexual and now considers herself a lesbian. She is out to everyone and even has her own YouTube video, "Gay Goddess." Julia doesn't care what people think of her sexual orientation. "It's their problem, and it's not for me to change their opinions."

Because Julia is so open, she has lost close friends—not everyone is as broadminded as her mother. One of Julia's schoolmates called her "disgusting" and was sent to the guidance counselor at Julia's school, which has a zero-tolerance policy for homophobia. However, later the bully backtracked and said, "I was just kidding," receiving no punishment. Julia has been verbally harassed at her Unitarian church, where there is only one other lesbian kid, who is not officially out.

At a religious camp three hours from Austin, Julia was accused of "forcing a gay agenda about herself and answering campers' questions about being gender queer." However, the camp didn't see it that way, as they were getting complaints from parents. The camp leaders did not proselytize and tell her she was sinful, although they did ask her a common question: "How do you know?"

Julia feels that the adults' reactions are worse than her contemporaries' and advises parents not to treat a gay child any differently than a straight child. She suggests that family therapy is a good idea and that the child or parent should first go alone. "Unload problems with the therapist, not the child. Don't add tension to the relationship."

If there is anything I've learned from straight parents interviewed for this book, it's that their love for their child eventually trumps their denial, guilt, fear, anger, shame, or loss.

It may take parents, through hard work, a while to arrive at acceptance of their child's sexuality. Some parents haven't reached acceptance—and they may never do so. Even if you, the reader, don't feel you've reached that goal, I applaud you for trying. You would not have read this book if you weren't seeking self-improvement.

Even I, after nineteen years of dealing with my own issues, always feel as if I could be doing more to edge toward greater acceptance of my son's sexuality, as I point out in the next chapter.

THE DOCTOR IS IN

Are you experiencing loss? If you agree with any of these statements, then you are probably struggling with loss:

- Having a gay son means I will never be a grandmother.
- I always imagined my daughter settling down with a nice man, but now I feel like I cannot imagine her future at all.
- Catholicism is the cornerstone of my life, and I feel lost and hopeless because I cannot seek comfort in my religion right now.
- If my son is gay, he is no longer welcome in this family.

As a psychiatrist, I frequently work with patients who are struggling with loss. The experience of loss is one that no one can avoid, for it is the great equalizer among us. Various life events can engender feelings of loss, such as divorce, job termination, terminal illness, and death. Following any significant loss, the normal emotional response usually takes the form of grief. The more significant the loss, the more severe the grief response will be. In 1969, the well-known psychiatrist Elisabeth Kübler-Ross devised a five-stage model of grief that originally described the experience of patients diagnosed with a terminal illness. Since that time, her model has been extrapolated to all forms of loss. The stages are denial, anger, bargaining, depression, and acceptance. Some of these stages are analogous to the phases that parents of a gay child may experience, which I describe elsewhere in this book. Although the majority of patients Kübler-Ross studied progressed through all five stages in a linear fashion, many did not. In some instances, people bypassed a stage or two, and in others, they occurred in varying orders. Some even skipped the first four stages altogether and immediately arrived at acceptance. Later in life, Kübler-Ross clarified her model, stating that there is "not a typical response to loss as there is no typical loss. Our grieving is as individual as our lives."

It is rare to work with parents of a gay child who have not struggled with the feeling of loss at some point in the process of accepting their child as gay. The most basic and common manifestation that I have come across is the loss of the type of life they envisioned for their child. When parents first learn the gender of their child, either during the pregnancy or upon delivery, they naturally begin to imagine what the child will be like and the trajectory his or her life will take. I have found that the content of these fantasies is consistent and often includes images of certain developmental milestones such as Little League games, dollhouses, prom dates, college graduations, and wedding days. Even in today's gender-progressive society, it is common for a man to conjure up visions of playing catch with his son and talking to him about dating girls, while a woman may fantasize about playing house with her daughter and taking her shopping one day for her wedding dress.

It is important to realize that the loss of this imagined life is not limited to parents of gay children but rather is a universal experience that parents of almost any child will face at some point. As I discussed in an earlier chapter, it is healthy, normal, and generally unavoidable for parents to have fantasies about their child's future. Furthermore, there is nothing wrong or unhealthy with a parent's attempt to cultivate these visions into actualized outcomes. However, it is also crucial that parents remain flexible in their ideas and, most importantly, that they are receptive to feedback, verbal and otherwise, from their child along the way.

For example, I worked with a teenage boy who had been taking piano lessons since he was four years old because his mother dreamed that he would be the next Beethoven. His mother was a piano virtuoso, who had never quite made it as a concert pianist and now worked in finance. My patient, however, did not share her vision. When he was young and had no autonomy, he complied with the daily lessons, initially basking in the praise and attention that his impressive talent earned him. However, as he entered adolescence, he preferred to spend his time in other ways. He had developed an interest in basketball and enjoyed shooting hoops with friends at his school gym in the afternoons instead of rushing home to a piano lesson. This caused tremendous strife between him and his mother. The conflict began to permeate the entire family as the boy's father felt torn between aligning with his wife and helping his son achieve the freedom and independence he deserved.

Parents must realize that their children are not extensions of themselves but, instead, are autonomous beings with their own set of dreams and hopes. I frequently work with families in crisis over a child's deviation from a parent's preconceived expectation. Take the case of parents who are distressed that their child does not wish to join and ultimately take over a business that has been in the family for generations. Rather than feel pride and admiration for their child who would rather forge her own path and cultivate a career for which she is passionate, parents feel rejection and disappointment. "How could she be so selfish and do this to us?" they wonder since they always "just assumed" that their daughter would take over the business. Parents are initially unable to reframe the situation in order to allow themselves to appreciate the noble qualities underlying their child's passion, which, ironically enough, they themselves likely inspired; instead, they are mired in the rigidity of their long-held notions. These situations require mental exercises involving identification with the other person and their perspective. Moreover, usually the parents need to do the real work in the therapy.

Although it may seem like we have detoured from parenting gay children to Parenting 101, rest assured that the case of a parent struggling with having a gay child is more similar to the preceding patient scenarios than you might initially realize. In both situations, there is a firmly held assumption and an emotional response that follows the realization that the child is not going to fulfill a preconceived wish. The vignettes involving a child forging his or her own unique career path are, in some ways, easier to negotiate. There is a concrete expectation of parents followed by a rational response from the child, clearly explaining why he or she would feel unfulfilled in the role desired by the parents. Conversely, gay parents often have a hard time elucidating the nature of the specific loss, stating something vague like, "It just wasn't the life I imagined for you," or "I always thought you'd have a regular family." My work with these parents always involves getting past the generalities and uncovering the specific losses that parents are truly grieving. Throughout these sessions, I have repeatedly come across three themes, which I will discuss and then propose how a parent can work through the loss.

Loss of a "Traditional Life"

The most common cause of distress experienced by parents of gay children is the notion that their child will not lead a "traditional life." By that, parents explain that they had a mental picture of their child's future that included a spouse, children, and family holidays. However, in our contemporary, pluralistic culture, it is becoming increasingly difficult to identify one uniform manifestation of a "traditional life," and I happen to think we are all better for it. Individuals choose to live their lives in myriad ways. My advice to parents, therefore, is to realize that it is not their place to impose specific life visions on their children. Again, this is not a message for parents of gay children only. In fact, I have worked with patients who are distraught upon learning that their *straight* son plans not to marry or their *straight* daughter is choosing not to have children. Moreover, my advice to these parents is no different from what I tell the parents of gay children. You do not get a vote in the major life decisions that your child makes. You should talk to your children, using neutral language that connotes curiosity, and ask them nonjudgmental questions so that you can understand how they have arrived at this important conclusion. Remember that your goal is not to change their minds or get them to "see the light" but simply for you to understand them better so that you can feel more connected to them.

In the case of gay children, when your child comes out to you, you should ask him how he envisions his life and what his dreams are. Let him speak freely without interjecting specific questions or stating assumptions. For example, many parents will say within the first five minutes of a child coming out to them, "So I guess I will never get to be a grandparent." However, you may be surprised to learn how "traditional" many gay teenagers envision their future to be. Over the last five years, a precipitous shift in public policy and constitutional law has made gay marriage legal in all fifty states. Moreover, adoption and surrogacy are becoming increasingly common as more gay people are looking to have children of their own. Nevertheless, although most parents of gay children are not ignorant of current events, many of them do not personally know anyone who is gay and married with children. As a result, they have a hard time making the leap from the abstract possibility to the concrete reality. Parents must realize that being gay does not necessarily mean a life of solitude and the absence of children, although it may. You should realize that your child might have rejected the institution of marriage whether he is gay or straight. Nevertheless, the larger message here is that being gay does not change or limit what your child can achieve, nor does it eliminate your obligation to stand by your child. Supporting your child as she makes major life decisions is a fundamental part of being a good parent. You should talk to your child to better understand her hopes and dreams and do whatever you can to help her achieve them.

Loss of an "Easy, Safe Life"

Most parents hope that their children will have an easier life than they had. By that, they generally mean smooth life trajectory with minimal hardship, conflict, and distress. Coming out as gay is a process associated with varying degrees of angst and emotional turmoil that most parents would not wish for their child to experience. Many parents with whom I have worked have said that they feel sad that their gay child has lost the possibility of having a life without significant difficulty. They come to me in a state of mourning, yet what they are actually grieving is the loss of their child's safety and innocence. They have arrived at this notion because the media frequently portrays gay struggles such as fights for equality, teenage bullying, and hate crimes. It is hard to disagree with a parent who sadly states, "But his life would be a lot easier if he weren't gay."

It is impossible to cocoon your child from every conceivable difficult circumstance he or she may encounter in life. Furthermore, even if you could somehow do that, it would not necessarily be a good thing. The challenging circumstances we face in our lives build character and give us strength. Our struggles not only define us, but they also contribute to our growth and development. If you speak with gay people who have been out of the closet for some time and ask them if they wish they had not been gay, in my experience, almost all of them would say no. When asked why, they state that they are happy with who they are and feel that they have emerged on the other side of coming out as strong, sensitive, and resilient individuals. As a parent, you, too, should embrace the challenge that having a gay child presents to you. How you choose to handle that challenge will be part of what defines your identity and your life.

Loss of a Child

Last, and thankfully, least common, is the notion that having a gay child is, in some way, a loss of the child altogether. When probed, parents who believe this reveal one of two things. First, they fear that being gay is in some way a death sentence for their child. While this may have been closer to reality in the 1970s and 1980s, being gay now does not automatically imply an HIV diagnosis and truncated lifespan.

Second, some parents feel that they will never be able to integrate this new information with their concept of their child, so their initial reaction is to reject the child altogether. I am sure you have all heard or read about a scenario in which a parent says something such as, "If you're gay, you are no longer my child." Or, "You can make a choice: Continue to be part of this family or be gay on your own." My advice to parents who jump to this conclusion upon learning that their child is gay is not to act on it right away. Disowning a child for any reason is a drastic and monumental move to make—one that should never be made without serious consideration involving a thorough and rigorous exploration of all possible alternatives. Once those words are spoken, it is very difficult to retract them. As I have said in previous chapters, there are always ways to repair a situation that was not handled in the best way initially, but telling a child she or he is no longer part of the family is perhaps the hardest one to remedy. The most common mistake parents make is conveying their unfiltered, negative emotions to their child at a critical time when they need to reaffirm their love and acceptance of their child. If you feel consumed by grief and anger, you should consult with a psychotherapist to help you figure out the best way to handle these complex emotions.

Parents of gay children struggle with loss in other forms. I have also worked with people who had a hard time reconciling their religious tenets with the newfound reality of their child's sexuality. In this socially progressive era, many religions have altered their official doctrine to varying degrees in support of gay rights. Although people integrate religion into their life for various reasons, most people affiliate with a religion and place of worship because it provides them with comfort and support, especially in the face of loss and crisis. If your religion is unable to do that for you during the time your child is coming out, then I suggest a couple of options. In almost all cases, I do not think it is necessary for someone to reject his or her current religion completely. If there is no one at your place of worship who can help you, one option is to find a clergyman at another place of worship who is more experienced and open-minded regarding homosexuality. People in every religion have found acceptable ways of modifying some of their beliefs to suit their particular situations or needs. I have had patients who remained as devout as they had always been but simply needed a change in their place of worship. For some, however, this might not be possible. If your religion unwaveringly shuns homosexuality and you still want to affiliate with that religion, I would recommend seeking support on this specific topic in other realms such as local PFLAG chapters and family support groups. Try as much as possible to compartmentalize this issue, keeping it out of your dealings with your place of worship, although I recognize that this may not always be easy or even feasible.

· 7 ·

ACCEPTANCE TO CELEBRATION

"The beginning of love is to let those we love be perfectly themselves and not to twist them to fit our own image."

—American author and mystic Thomas Merton (1915–1968)

THERE IS NO timetable for acceptance of a gay or lesbian child. The journey is a process and may entail working through the stages described in the previous chapters at your own speed. However you demonstrate acceptance, it should be at your own comfort level. Don't judge yourself! The themes of these chapters only illustrate what is *possible*.

Even I, like the eighty-year-old mother in Chapter 3, dislike gay parades. I find the nearly naked, thong-wearing men I see on Gay Pride floats unpleasant, so I tend to avoid the parades. (For that matter, so does my son!) But at the same time, I admire gay activists like Katy Bourne (see page 100) who rides in a carriage with her gay son during Pride parades. We all discover the best ways—for our children and for ourselves—to show support.

I often feel guilty because I don't write senators about antidiscriminatory laws that should be passed. Later in this chapter, Dr. Tobkes suggests that a parent "talk to other family members and friends openly about your child being gay." I am still working on this. I am proud of my son, but if I feel chafed against the smallness of someone's religion, or if I know I'm going to feel as if I'm being judged for having a gay son, I don't volunteer that information. Nor do I discuss his dating life, even though I'm usually happy to chat about our daughter's boyfriends.

However, as I wrote in the acknowledgments, I feel more sensitive to the trials and tribulations of minorities, considering other perspectives at length where I would have otherwise accepted a simple explanation, or not thought about marginalized groups at all. I regard having a gay child as a "gift," a *raison d'être* for growth. Having a gay child is a chance to be an ally of a world in which I would not have been privileged to enter otherwise. It forces you out of your complacency as a parent and requires that you revise your relationship. A healthy relationship between a straight parent and a gay child can result in greater honesty and closeness. I've found that to be the case in my own life.

Although this chapter is about acceptance—and more—I am also including gay and lesbian adults who have dealt with parents who have refused to accept their lifestyles, which has produced dire effects. However, it's never too late, as Dr. Tobkes illustrates, for parents to apologize and try again to earn the respect and trust of their child.

One such individual who was not accepted for her sexual orientation is Heather Purser, who learned the hard way what parents should *not* do after their child comes out.

Heather Purser, Daughter, Thirty-Three

Heather lives in Seattle and works for a seafood company. She dives for clams called geoducks. She realized she was a lesbian at age seven. "There was a movie that had a gay character," she explained, "and my older sister explained what *gay* meant. And it clicked for me—I mean it really clicked. I knew I didn't quite fit in with everyone else but learned there were some other people in the world who didn't either."

She officially came out at age sixteen. It was no picnic. Her mother, with whom she no longer has contact, found a story that Heather had been writing. It would be classified today on a bookshelf as "lesbian romantic fiction." Rather than admiring Heather's creativity, her mother screamed at her and threw her down the stairs.

Then her mother assembled the rest of the family—two sisters and two brothers—and read aloud the juicy parts of Heather's story about two girls who met and kissed sometimes (the author's secret wish). As if that wasn't enough humiliation, Heather's mother then called all of their extended family members and told them to watch their children around Heather, as if Heather was going to molest them! Heather's mother warned them to check their computers after Heather had left their house to make sure there was no child pornography on file.

Heather's father, a fisherman, was absent quite a bit and admitted that he forgot Heather was gay every time she brought the subject up. The discrimination continued at college, where Heather was shunned for being *different*, not for being a lesbian but for being a very pale Native American woman. A quarter Native American of the Suquamish tribe, Heather has very fair skin and red hair. The only semblance of her father's native heritage is her high cheekbones.

After she was jumped and beaten in her dorm room, Heather transferred to Western Washington University in Willingham, where she came out again and found a better reception, especially with the other gay students. She graduated from WWU in 2009.

It was Heather's love for graduate student Rebecca Platter, to whom she is now engaged, as well as the concern for other gays and lesbians, that led to her decision to propose same-sex marriage at the Suquamish Tribe's annual council. "Suquamish are very live and let live—very progressive," she remarks. A year after Heather worked up the nerve to go and ask council members what they thought of same-sex marriage, she attended an open-floor council meeting. She stood up and stated again that she wanted support for same-sex marriage because she "felt not enough was happening and wanted to be more public." At first, the tribe was cautious, because it wanted to see if the Coquille Tribe, which had approved marriage equality, would experience any repercussions. Her tribe was reluctant to vote against the U.S. Supreme Court when it came to a ruling about gay marriage, as well.

Fortunately, that March, the tribe voted a resounding "Yes!" It was a vote that supported her desire to be able to marry another woman. The Suquamish Tribe is the first jurisdiction in the state of Washington to recognize same-sex marriage. It was set in stone in June 2012 as part of the tribe's constitution. For her foresight and activism, Heather was awarded the Seattle Human Rights Commission's Human Rights Award in 2011.

Despite Heather's accomplishments, her family continued to regard her sexual orientation as an embarrassment. "My mother and sisters took it to be their burden. It isn't their drama," warns Heather. "Being gay is not about them. It's about *me*, but it *becomes* their problem when they don't accept me. They should have reassured me that they loved me."

While a parent may regard a child's sexual orientation as a funeral procession for his hopes and dreams for that child, experiencing a deep sense of loss, Heather is quick to point out that it is also a loss for the child. "Parents should remember that their children want to fit into society; being gay does not make you blend in."

Although Mitchel Bauer has not suffered from the physical abuse that Heather has, he has felt, and still feels, the sting of parental rejection from his parents for being gay.

Mitchel Bauer, Son, Twenty-Five

Mitchel Bauer is every parent's dream of an ideal son. Growing up on a farm that originally belonged to his grandfather in Snelling, California, Mitchel was an all-around great child. He was a bright pupil who was homeschooled by his mother, and he helped care for her seven other children. He obediently did chores on the farm, which sells organic chickens and almonds. His parents inculcated a strong work ethic in him that he never resented. If he wanted to earn extra money, he asked for extra chores on the farm and was paid a minimum wage.

He was also a good athlete and played on basketball and football teams at a Christian school nearby. The son of evangelical Christians, he spent many hours in church and with youth groups.

When Mitchel was a senior in the fall of 2007, he wrote a three-page letter to his parents about the fact that he had same-sex attractions and felt confused, although he never labeled himself "gay." He received no response from them. A couple of weeks went by—still no response. Mitchel brought the letter up again and was still ignored.

While at Merced Community College, he met his future wife, Sarah. They were at a Campus Crusade for Christ meeting for a sermon on life's struggles. Mitchel was asked to pick a card and write down his personal struggle. He wrote "homosexuality."

Sarah saw the card. Nevertheless, despite Mitchel's strong attraction to men, he married Sarah, whom he found to be "open, honest, and genuine," when he was twenty-one. She was the only girl he ever dated. The marriage lasted over three years, and the subsequent divorce resulted in a deep depression for Mitchel.

He thought he was separating from Sarah as a stepping-stone to divorce; she thought they were separating to fix the marriage. She was hurt that he wanted men more than her and that he had affairs with them. For Mitchel, he felt guilty that he couldn't change and that he was getting divorced even though he still loved his wife. He felt like a loser and a failed Christian.

The same-sex attractions never lessened as he hoped they would. He kept rationalizing that his sexuality didn't define him. But it did, and he ended up in the hospital for depression.

During that time, his older sister, Patricia, who acted as his confidante *in loco parentis*, stressed to their parents that Mitchel was in "crisis mode." He reached out to his parents, who told him to get counseling and that he had *chosen* to live "a sinful life." They recommended that he "come back to the church" and renew his relationship with his wife.

Mitchel's parents are embarrassed that he has since announced his new identity, via e-mails and phone calls, to various members of the family. The reaction in his church back home is almost identical to what it was when he was eighteen: At that time, he was told to get married, as, according to them, the practice of homosexuality is sinful.

Mitchel feels as if his parents have abandoned him. He is not allowed home for Christmas, and he is forbidden from contacting the younger siblings who used to admire him, because his parents think he might put homosexual thoughts in their heads.

Patricia, who lives in San Diego, calls her brother regularly to stay in touch. She is genuinely concerned about him. "My parents should reach out to him," she commented. "He's had a huge lifestyle change. He's working three jobs (Starbucks, Old Navy, and Roadhouse Grill), doesn't have a car, and has little family contact."

Mitchel has found the gay community in Harrisburg, Pennsylvania, where he lives, to be very supportive. They give him rides to work and job leads. He seems to be relieved to be out of the closet.

"My parents need time," says Patricia. "It's hard for them to accept his new identity. We're a close family, so maybe they'll come around. They could call him just to say hi and not play the gay card. . . . Love the sinner, but not the sin?'"

Two weeks ago, however, Patricia saw some glacial progress with Mitchel's parents. Their father has a habit of e-mailing his children and telling them he loves them and to have a good day. In the past, Mitchel has received just a biblical message alluding to homosexuality, separate from his siblings. On this particular day, Patricia noticed that Mitchel was included in the family's group e-mail with the message, "Love you, have a good day!"—no Bible verse.

Next month, Mitchel will see his father when he attends his younger sister's college graduation in Alabama. While he and his father have not plumbed the subject of his same-sex attraction, the fact that his father has dropped the biblical references in his e-mails to Mitchel is an auspicious start.

Some gay and lesbian children are lucky to have accepting parents from the get-go. Such is Walker Vreeland.

Walker Vreeland, Son, Thirty-Seven

A popular Long Island, New York, radio personality, Walker Vreeland has won numerous awards at his station, 102.5 WBAZ-FM. Walker is openly gay, on and off the radio. He would probably not be as self-confident in his sexuality if it were not for his accepting family.

As a host and producer, Walker uses his own autobiographical material in which he is candid about his past struggles with his sexuality despite a very accepting family, as well as his history of mental illness. "What lies beneath everything I do on the air is a fundamental desire to make people feel less alone in the world. Is that desire to connect somehow related to the loneliness I experienced growing up gay?" philosophizes Walker.

For his radio work, he was voted Best Media Personality in the Hamptons in 2013, 2014, and 2015. With a graduate degree in broadcasting from the prestigious Tisch School for the Arts at New York University, Walker had appeared in plays, television, and film. But it is radio where he feels more secure with the sharing, the interviews, and *his* writing.

Walker came out to his mother first when he was a senior in high school. She was not surprised, although he had a girlfriend in his sophomore year, which confused her. Fortunately for Walker, she didn't doubt him by responding, as many parents do, by saying, "How could you be gay? You had a girlfriend," or maybe, "It's just a phase!" Says Walker, "Sexuality can be fluid, and just because your son had a girlfriend last year, and even appeared to be genuinely interested in her, that doesn't necessarily mean that he is straight if he is now telling you that he is gay. Parents should know better than to doubt."

He continues that a parent should tell their son or daughter, "I love you for who you are." This is unconditional love, what every gay or lesbian child desires. Otherwise, the relationship will suffer, and, as Walker has seen with his contemporaries, the child will look elsewhere for a support system.

However, as Walker comments, if a parent doesn't react well to the child's coming out, it's important not to shame the child. It's okay for parents to admit that they are working on their own issues, not the son's or daughter's! If possible, parents should seek advice from a gay friend who can educate them or a close straight friend or relative who won't be judgmental, as Dr. Tobkes has made clear in previous chapters.

As parents are not given a handbook for raising gay and lesbian children, they shouldn't be expected to know how to parent a gay or lesbian child while, at the same time, trying to adjust their own expectations. As gay San Francisco columnist Dan Savage of *Savage Love* counsels, "If you, as a parent, need to take a couple of years to process, that's fine. But if after that time, you still can't accept your child, understand that they might well move on in search of unconditional love elsewhere."

Like Walker, John Paul Brammer was accepted by his family, but certainly not by his peers in middle school.

John Paul Brammer, Son, Twenty-Four

When he was in parochial school near Lawton, Oklahoma, John Paul Brammer didn't know he was gay. He *did* know he had crushes on male classmates as far back as the first grade.

He later switched to public middle school to be closer to home. Unfortunately, his new school made him miserable. His friends, whose parents were in the military, moved away. He was depressed, gained a lot of weight, and on top of that, realized he was gay in the sixth grade. So did the other kids, who teased him because of his mannerisms.

John wouldn't admit his secret to anyone. He told his parents that he wanted to commit suicide. His grades were slipping. Still, he wouldn't reveal his sexual orientation. After all, his father made homophobic remarks at the television, and his mother, Hispanic, was raised Catholic. He didn't want to disappoint them, and he was ashamed.

That *big* secret stayed with him until he was twenty and away at the University of Oklahoma (OU) working on a journalism degree. Today, he lives in Washington, D.C., and writes for *The Blue Nation Review*, *The Advocate*, *Huffington Post/Gay Voices*, as well as *BuzzFeed*, *Remezela*, and *Vox*. John writes on LGBT and Latino issues and is a gay rights activist.

He came out in a casual way. A friend of his was showing him a picture of her boyfriend, who John said he found attractive. The friend was a member of the Sooner Allies at the university—folks who have been trained to provide resources and support for LGBT and questioning members of the OU community. "I was testing the waters," admitted John. "Suddenly, I felt different admitting that I was gay. I was exhilarated!" After taking that first step of coming out, he felt more confident to tell other people.

Finally, on the first day of his junior year in college, he told his parents when his father asked him to look out for his sister, an incoming freshman at the same college.

However, he told his sister that he was bisexual so she wouldn't think he was gay all those years. It helped him not to feel guilty about his cover-up. She was fine with the notion, but a month or two later, John told her the actual truth.

John's parents were accepting. His mother was not surprised, and his father told him just what he wanted to hear—that he loved him. That summer, John fell hard for a boy who wasn't out of the closet. That boy's father broke up the relationship between his son and John.

When John came out, his mother asked him if he had known he was gay in middle school, during the worst years of his depression. She apologized for the unsafe atmosphere she had contributed to during those years. "Because she put her pride first," John says, "and knew so many people in their rural community who might gossip," she had told John not to announce his suicidal ideation!

"When you are coming out, it's not a good time for the other person to interject their thoughts" commented John. "It means you're not listening, and it stops the whole sexuality discussion in its tracks, so the focus is on the parent, not the person who is coming out." When a child comes out, the parent shouldn't respond with questions, cautions John. It gives the impression to the child that you're not listening to this important revelation but only somehow want to relate it to how it is going to affect your life, not the child's.

John's other tip for parents is that they should not change the subject when a gay or lesbian child talks about his or her same-sex significant other. "They may say they are accepting, but their actions say otherwise. It's as if they accept but then don't want to talk about it. It's a double standard, because they don't do this with their heterosexual child."

Every child dreams of the perfect time and place for coming out. Although Tanner Hockey's mother was accepting, the coming out was not the right venue, and this left him resentful.

Tanner Hockey, Son, Eighteen

Tanner, a student studying fashion marketing at The Art Institute of Vancouver, British Columbia, relayed that he has had a relatively easy time being gay. In the creative world, there is a much more liberal setting for LGBT people. He also lives in Canada, which legalized same-sex marriage in 2005—way before the United States!

The only "bumps" in the road, as he calls them, seemed to be in elementary school. He knew he was *different*, as many gay men and women do, because of the way he dressed. But at the time he thought being *gay* meant you had long hair.

He bought skinny jeans in the fifth grade. In high school, he wore really short shorts with slits, which were deemed to be inappropriate attire, and he was sent home by the principal. Tanner laughed it off. He commented, "I wanted a handbag desperately, but my mother thought it was just too feminine and forbade me to own one."

The same-sex attraction started around sixth grade. Two friends in the eighth grade knew he was gay. Tanner was not interested in sports, but he liked drawing in high school.

The first person he told he was gay was his older sister, age twenty-two, whom he lives with now. She in turn relayed the news to their mother. Tanner was miffed that *he* never came out to his mother on his own terms. "My mother thought I was depressed and could be on drugs and was having 'a really hard time,'" he said. "She was not surprised at the news, but she didn't have to tell other members of the family. That was my job!" Luckily, Tanner was accepted by his entire family, including the conservative ones.

After he came out, Tanner felt relief, but he was surprised that not everything got better right away. He finds Gay Pride Day an excuse to get drunk, as do some observers of St. Patrick's Day in Manhattan. He also sees that the younger generation, of which he is a part, forgets that the same-sex equality was fought for by the older generation.

"Of course, life is always easier when you're not a member

of a minority group. There could be discrimination at a job even though, since the mid-nineties, sexual orientation was included in the Canadian Human Rights Act and protected in the Equal Rights Section of the Charter 1."

Tanner believes if acceptance isn't going well, it could be for these three reasons: First, "if a father is struggling with understanding the definition of 'masculinity,' and what it means now that he knows his son is gay, it is important for the father to realize that the son is still the same person. Being gay doesn't mean you're less of a 'man.'"

Second, according to Tanner, having a gay child can sometimes embarrass the parent, possibly because of her social group. Outside opinions don't define the relationship between parent and child, and they shouldn't affect it. Parents should ignore the unwanted advice of outsiders.

Third, "many parents, says Tanner, "are worried about AIDS/HIV based on outdated information. The virus is prevalent, but it's not the eighties when gay people were dying of what amounted to a plague. Parents should know that HIV is under control now with drugs and is not considered the death sentence it was years ago." (Nevertheless, parents should talk and continue to talk about using condoms to prevent the disease in the first place.)

Briana Popour is nearly the same age as Tanner. Even though she lives in a less gay-accepting place than Canada, she has a more devil-may-care attitude in her home in Chesnee, South Carolina.

Briana Popour, Daughter, Nineteen

Briana knows her way around a school. Last year, she took a girl as her date to a prom. She also walked down the hallowed halls of Chesnee High School holding hands with a girl. She wore a T-shirt that says "Nobody knows I'm a Lesbian," and no one commented. This year, it was a different story.

One year later, the same T-shirt set off a controversy that was reported as far away as England. She received Facebook messages of congratulation from around the world. *The U.S. News & World Report* and *Washington Blade* wrote her up.

Administrators in her small school of 900 students pulled her out of class in September for wearing the T-shirt, now considered "distracting" to students and faculty. She was told either to go home and change the shirt or not return to school. Briana stood her ground.

She spoke up for herself and said, "There is nothing in the handbook about sexual orientation." Her mother supported her right to wear the shirt and said that an attorney contacted them the next day.

Now Briana only speaks to the principal through a lawyer. Even with a 4.0 average in some of her classes, she has teachers who give her a rough time, still singling her out. To them, she's a "troublemaker." To others, she's a bit of a hero. Briana's mother said the administrator "doesn't like people in high school wearing anything that says anything about LGB."

Briana told the school that they had no right not to let her wear the T-shirt. Briana, who has been attracted to women since elementary school, says, "You should be happy who you are. Isn't that what school is supposed to teach you? It's an identity. I and the other gay teens shouldn't be afraid." She is much happier being out and living an open and honest life.

She is typical of an ever-increasing number of gay, lesbian, and transgender children who are challenging their outmoded school dress codes so they can express their identity in a confident manner. Proud of who they are, they won't put up with stereotypical boy-girl proms or the ideology of old-fashioned school officials. They, like Briana, know their rights.

More than two years ago, Briana came out to her mother. "I hid it for a long time— even dated guys for fear I would be rejected," confessed Briana. "I was afraid of judgmental relatives." But she has found even her ninety-one-year-old grandmother to be more than accepting. In fact, when her grandmother was told the news, she remarked, "I could have told you that." Her cousin in Illinois sent Briana a T-shirt that reads "gay, bisexual, straight, and human" with boxes beside each identity. Her aunt says she is proud of her. "I wanted all of them to think highly of me," says Briana.

Briana's mother said she just wants her daughter to be happy. She doesn't care who her daughter dates as long as she is treated with respect, unlike the school's treatment of her daughter. Briana comments, "Remember that your child is still the same child, whether gay or straight. Love him; support her. One day, you will need [your children] to take care of you."

THE DOCTOR IS IN

Are you experiencing accweptance? If you agree with any of these statements, then you are probably approaching acceptance:

1. I truly don't care if my child is straight, gay, or bisexual. My only concern is that he is happy.
2. I love my child for who she is, and her sexuality doesn't change that.
3. I don't see a distinction between my daughter's husband and my son's husband. They are both my sons-in-law, and I am thankful that they make my children so happy.
4. I feel grateful that my child is lesbian because we have a closeness that I am not sure we could have achieved if she were straight.

Acceptance involves acknowledging the reality of a particular situation and recognizing that it is not in your power to change it. When faced with circumstances that are not only distressing but also unchangeable, the only way to alleviate internal angst and achieve a sense of equanimity is through acceptance. People often mistake tolerance for acceptance. For example, when a man marries a woman of a different faith, his parents might welcome their daughter-in-law into their family but still hold onto their belief that Catholics should not inter-marry and continue to feel that it would have been preferable if their son had married a Catholic. On the other hand, if they were to *accept* their son's decision, they might demonstrate this by embracing their daughter-in-law's religious traditions and using holiday celebrations, for instance, as a means of uniting their two families more deeply. Acceptance, in its most basic form, means not resisting reality and acknowledging that an event occurred and is real.

Acceptance of your gay child is often a gradual process that evolves over time, beginning with simply accepting that your child is definitively and permanently gay, that is, not thinking it is a phase or a choice; this is the most basic form of accep-tance. Accepting this reality is a crucial component of moving forward and developing an honest relationship with your child. If you cannot internalize the concept that your child is gay, and always will be, it will be quite difficult to cultivate a meaningful relationship with him. To the best of my knowledge, no child has ever "stopped being gay" because his family was not willing to accept it.

A more advanced level of acceptance is one in which you do not feel a qualitative difference between your straight child and your gay child. By this, I don't mean that you do not com-prehend that one child is heterosexual and the other homo-sexual but rather that you don't harbor biases or preferences toward the straight child. Parents should not prefer one child to another for any reason, but this is an elusive ideal that many parents do not achieve. I have worked with families in which parents say they are "totally fine" with the fact that their child is gay, but I often observe unmistakable differences between the way they act toward their gay child and their other children. For example, one patient reported that her mother put a lot of effort into making plans, such as lunch dates and museum outings, with her brother's wife, but never once did her mother do that with her own wife. When confronted with this discrepancy, her mother initially provided flimsy explanations like, "Wanda is vegan, and I wouldn't even know where to take her," or "I just can't get Wanda's schedule down." When pressed, however, she ultimately conceded that she wasn't making an equal effort to cultivate this relationship but couldn't explain why. Once this was brought to her attention, however, she genuinely felt bad; she apologized and said that she was willing to work on it. In my experience, most parents exhibiting this type of rejecting behavior are not doing so consciously or intentionally.

The ultimate level of acceptance that I have seen in a small subset of parents is to become a gay rights activist by doing such things as marching in Gay Pride parades and working toward effecting change through legislation. You should by no means feel the need to achieve this outcome, nor should your child put pressure on you to do these things. You should recognize that many gay people themselves do not feel it is necessary to be a crusader for gay rights. I am somewhat reluctant to include this for fear that people might think that if they do not arrive here, they have not successfully completed the acceptance process. Such is not the case.

If you are reading this book after reacting negatively to your child's coming out, you should realize that it is never too late to remedy the situation. Although you cannot retract your initial words, you can engage with your child in a dialogue with the purpose of understanding his coming-out experience better. For example, you might say something like, "What you told me last week really came as a surprise to me. While it may take me some time to digest this news, I hope you know that I will always love you, no matter what." You should also ask your child details about his coming-out experience and exhibit genuine interest. Interestingly, I have found in my practice that the process of acceptance that a child has been through often mirrors the process that a parent will go through, the only difference being that the child is further along on the journey. Talk to your child in a non-threatening manner, using "I" statements to express the way you are feeling, and give her your full attention. Be sure to initiate such a conversation at a time when you can speak without distractions or time constraint. It is okay to tell your child that you are working toward acceptance but are not there yet and hope to be soon. It is better to acknowledge that you are aware of your struggle for acceptance and are actively working toward it than to say nothing at all.

Although you may not have yet arrived at a state of true acceptance, there are still things you can and should do to provide your child with the comfort and stability that are crucial in leading to a positive outcome. This represents the "getting your lines right" component of the process. In other words, you can say the right things even if you are not yet fully at peace with the situation. Not only will this send a reassuring message to your child that you are unequivocally on his side, but it will also help you with your own acceptance. Here are some examples of things you can do or say to convey acceptance even if you are not fully there yet:

Ask your child the same questions you ask your other children. Specifically, don't avoid the topic of dating and relationships.

Ironically, most straight children find questions about their romantic life meddlesome and annoying, but they are generally a requisite part of the parent-child dynamic; by avoiding them with your gay child, you are treating him differently. One straight sibling joked to her gay brother, "I wish I were gay so mom would stop bugging me about getting married." This comment, although benign in its intention, was hurtful to her brother because it brought to the surface the feeling that his mother seemed less invested in him and his future happiness. If your gay child says that he is dating someone in particular, ask engaging questions about the partner and express an interest in meeting him. Be sure to invite the boyfriend to family dinners or functions in the same way you would for a partner of your straight child. From time to time, make a point of asking your child how his boyfriend is doing, what is new with him, and so forth.

Talk to other family members and friends openly about your child being gay, and share the same information you would with them about his dating life as you would about your straight child.

If you are initially having a hard time saying, "Judy is a lesbian," it may be more comfortable for you to start out saying something like, "Judy dates women," or "Judy has a girlfriend." Many parents with whom I have worked admit that they are very quick to tell their friends when their straight daughter has a new boyfriend but are reluctant to discuss their gay son's dating life and relationships. Avoidance of these topics with your close confidantes presents a major roadblock on the path to acceptance.

You should make a point of talking to your child about how he wants to handle letting relatives and close family friends know.

By the time children tell their parents they are gay, the vast majority of them have already achieved their own personal acceptance of the reality of their sexuality. In many cases, they have told their close friends or are even "out" at school. Coming out to their extended family, however, often presents a significant challenge to gay youth, and it is, therefore, an opportunity for you to ally with your child and demonstrate your acceptance. I have seen cases in which the child wants the autonomy of telling each person himself and, more commonly, situations in which he wants them to know but is not particularly interested in having each individual conversation. You should ask an open-ended question such as, "Have you thought about how and when you want to tell Grandma?" Your child may respond with something such as, "Not really. Do you think you could just let everyone know for me?" You should defer to your child on how he wants to handle informing the other important people in your family's life. Most importantly, you should in no way imply that he should keep it a secret from certain people or act as if he should feel embarrassed or ashamed for other people to know. If your child expresses concern about telling a particular relative, you can then engage in a conversation in which you explore the merits and potential consequences of telling a staunchly conservative grandfather, for example. However, the hesitation should never come from you because your child may perceive it as a projection of your own tacit disapproval or shame.

In my work with families, there have been certain concepts that have repeatedly emerged that have helped a parent move closer to radical acceptance. Here are three such realizations that parents have had at various points along their journeys that I hope are helpful to you, too.

It is worthwhile for parents to recognize the qualities in their child that may not have been present if he were straight.

I hate to subscribe to clichés or stereotypes, but, for example, there is something to the notion that gay sons are often more emotionally connected to their mothers than are straight sons. A woman with whom I worked had always appreciated her shared interests and frequent heart-to-heart conversations with her son. When he came out to her, she initially could not accept it, saying that he "wasn't who [she] thought he was," and she worried that they wouldn't be close anymore because he was "a different person now." Upon reflection, however, she came to the realization that perhaps the converse was true, that is, they were close *because* he was gay. Her son's ability to connect easily and deeply with his mother is a quality that is probably linked to his sexuality. She ultimately realized that he had always been gay, just as he was always thoughtful and compassionate, and that she loved him for who he was regardless of his sexuality. She stated, "I now realize that it's not possible to pick and choose qualities in a person as if you're picking a meal from an à la carte menu. You cannot expect to change one trait and not have others change with it."

In other situations, parents have felt that there was always something preventing them from achieving a sense of closeness with their child; however, when their child came out to them, they connected with him in ways that they didn't know were possible. "It was like there was a giant wall that I couldn't even see, but upon coming out to me, it just crumbled in a single instant," said one parent. Almost all parents with whom I have worked have definitely felt that their relationship with their child was qualitatively better than it was before their child came out to them. Moreover, the achievement of a deeper relationship led them not only to accept their child's sexuality but also to appreciate it because of that newfound closeness.

Parents who consider that having a happy child is more important than having a child who fits a certain mold are more likely to accept having a gay child than those who hold firmly to preconceived beliefs.

At the end of the day, an ideal parent is one who prioritizes his or her child's happiness, as trite as that may seem. If your child is gay and at peace with it, you should feel content and relieved that he is not struggling to accept his sexuality, and, therefore, you yourself should not indulge in a struggle to accept it.

Last, some parents are able to take a step back, see the larger picture, and realize that there can be personal benefits to having a gay child.

One parent pointed out to me that having a child who is in a minority group has made him more sensitive to others who are struggling for acceptance and equality. Another mother said that she has become more open-minded and less likely to make snap judgments of others or participate in petty gossip. Most experiences in our life are opportunities for personal growth if we are willing to reflect and find the deeper meaning in them. You should use this experience of being the parent of a gay child as a catalyst not only for deepening your relationship with your child but also for examining the way you conceptualize society.

As I have stated earlier, a key variable in determining a positive outcome—one without drugs, violence, mental illness, or HIV—for a gay individual is the perception of his or her family's acceptance. Even if you are just beginning your journey toward acceptance, my final message is that you can and should demonstrate to your child *in both words and actions* that you will always love and support him or her unconditionally. Doing so will keep the lines of communication open between you and your child so that you can gain a better understanding of your child's sexuality and ultimately arrive at true acceptance of it.

Endnotes

Foreword

xi   **The statistics are chilling:** "LGBT Youth Statistics," Project Q, accessed December 11, 2015, http://www.endabusewi.org /sites/default/files/resources/lgbt_youth_facts_and_stats.pdf.

xi   **What is even more terrifying:** Ibid.

xi   **But there is a bright side:** "Accepting Parents Boost Health of LGBT Teens," Jeanna Bryner, accessed December 11, 2015, http://www.livescience.com/9075-accepting-parents -boost-mental-health-lgbt-teens.html.

Chapter 1

21   **Ashlee, an assistant at a midsize publishing company:** Oregon's now governor Kate Brown, former Oregon secretary of state, is the highest ranking bisexual public official in U.S. history. She was told by her parents, "It would be much easier for us if you were a lesbian." During her campaign, she was told to "butch it up." She is married to a man, Dan Little, a U.S. Forest Service data expert. Samantha Allen, "Bisexuality's Watershed Political Moment," *The Daily Beast*, February 14, 2015, https://www.thedailybeast.com /articles/2015/02/14/bisexuality-s-watershed-political -moment.html.

21   **Despite her confirmation as a bisexual:** Over the past year,
     approximately 800,000 people updated their profile to include
     same-gender attraction or entered a custom gender. This
     figure is three times what it was a year ago, according to a
     report from Facebook's Research and Data Science division.
     Alyssa Newcomb, "Facebook Reveals More People Than Ever
     Are Coming Out on the Social Network," *ABCNews.go.com*,
     October 16, 2015, http://abcnews.go.com/Technology
     /facebook-reveals-people-coming-social-network/story?id
     = 34525189.

Chapter 2

36   **I no longer believe, as:** The most influential source of the
     "absent father/overprotective mother" theory of
     homosexuality was a research project conducted by
     psychoanalyst Irving Bieber, author of *Homosexuality: A
     Psychoanalytic Study of Male Homosexuals* (New York: Basic
     Books, 1962). His conclusion was that male homosexuality is
     caused by "paternal hostility and engulfing maternalism."
     Mothers of gay men were found to be seductive, babying, and
     controlling. Fathers were distant, competitive, or hostile.
     Despite the fact that Bieber's conclusions were repudiated by
     mainstream psychology and psychiatry decades ago, Christian
     reparative (pray-the-gay-away, or conversion therapy)
     continues to cite his studies in support of their treatment.

37   **Despite the growing body:** WebMD, "Is There a Gay
     Gene?," accessed December 4, 2015, http://www.webmd.com
     /sex-relationships/news/20050128/is-there-gay-gene.
     Researchers say it's the first time the entire human genetic
     makeup has been scanned in search of possible genetic
     determinants of male sexual orientation. The results suggest
     that several genetic regions may influence homosexuality.

Chapter 3

70   **If he hadn't known about how:** One of the biggest studies on the experiences of transgender people was the 2011 *National Transgender Discrimination Survey (NTDS)*. It found that in the United States, 41 percent of transgender and gender nonconforming people had attempted suicide, compared to a national average of just 4.6 percent. Zack Ford, "No, High Suicide Rates Do Not Demonstrate That Transgender People Are Mentally Ill," ThinkProgress.org, June 22, 2015, https://www.thinkprogress.org/lgbt /2015/06/. . . /transgender-suicide-rate.

70   **As enthusiastic as he was:** The legal age in the United States for adolescents and young adults diagnosed with transsexualism is eighteen. "Care of the Child with the Desire to Change Genders," *Medscape*, 2010, www.medscape.com /viewarticle/722004_2.

71   **He has not yet had:** Gender reassignment surgery (GRS) is terribly expensive, costing up to $100,000, usually out-of -pocket, and is irreversible. Many transgender people do not elect to do GRS because of the expense. Alyssa Jackson, "The High Cost of Being Transgender," CNN.com, July 31, 2015, https://www.cnn.com/2015/07/31/health/transgender-costs -irpt/.

71   **When he was a summer intern:** Colorado is a state that protects against both sexual orientation and gender identity discrimination in employment in the private and public sector. However, in approximately half of the United States an employer can legally fire a LGBT person in the workplace. Wikipedia.org, accessed February 12, 2016, https:// en.wikipedia.org/wiki/LGBT_employment_discrimination _in_the_United States.

74 **He and his wife worried:** At this writing, in the majority of states, there are no protections against discrimination based on your sexual orientation. There has been legislation introduced to amend the Civil Rights Act of 1964 to add sexual orientation and gender identity to the list of already protected classes.

77 **In addition, the use of pre-exposureprophylaxis:** Tim Horn, "PrEP in iPrEx: 92% Fewer Infections in Those with Detectable Drug Levels," AIDSmeds.com, July 22, 2011, http://www.aidsmeds.com/articles/hiv_prep _iprex_2636_20876.shtml

80 **Many studies have demonstrated the increased risk:** Jerome Hunt, "Why the Gay and Transgender Population Experiences Higher Rates of Substance Use," Center for American Progress, March 9, 2012, https://www .americanprogress.org/issues/lgbt/report/w2012/03/09/11228 /why-the-gay-and-transgender-population-experiences -higher-rates-of-substance-use/.

82 **Of all the hate crimes reported annually:** "Latest Hate Crime Statistics Report Released," FBI.org, December 8, 2014, https://www.fbi.gov/news/stories/2014/december /latest-hate-crime-statistics-report-released.

Chapter 5

115 **At that point, she was:** A *New York Times* article from October 15, 2015, "Outgrowing 'Tomboy'" by Marisa Meltzer, says, "'tomboy' is a term now deemed old-fashioned with new phrases like 'gender nonconformist' taking its place."

116 **After ten months, she decided:** This law banning gays in military was repealed on September 20, 2011.

117 **Sometimes I do feel bad:** This would not be true today. As of June 26, 2015, the Supreme Court legalized same-sex marriage throughout the United States in a 5-4 landmark decision.

Chapter 6

151 **Many studies have demonstrated:** See Jerome Hunt, "Why the Gay and Transgender Population Reports Higher Rates of Substance Use," American Progress, accessed December 4, 2015, https://www.americanprogress.org/issues/lgbt /report/2012/ 03/09/11228/why-the-gay-and-transgender -population-experiences-higher-rates-of-substance-use.

159 **Later in life, Kübler-Ross:** Elizabeth Kübler-Ross and David Kessler, *On Grief and Grieving*, Simon & Schuster, 2005.

Resources for Straight Families and LGBT Adults

For Families and Friends

Family Acceptance Project: Cesar E. Chavez Institute, San Francisco
    State University
familyproject.sfsu.edu
e-mail: fap@sfsu.edu

The Parents Project
www.theparentsproject.com

PFLAG
www.pflag.org

Videos

Mosbacher, Dee, *Straight from the Heart: Parents' Journeys to Under-
    standing and Love of their Gay and Lesbian Children*, Woman Vision
    Video, 1994. This documentary explores the relationships between
    straight parents and gay children.

Anti-Bullying

Gay-Straight Alliance
www.gsa.org

GLSEN (Gay, Lesbian Straight Educational Network)
www.glsen.org

Safe Schools Coalition
www.safeschoolscoalition.org

Stop Bullying
www.stopbullying.gov

Bisexual Resources and Transgender Resources

BiNet USA. An advocacy organization specifically for bisexuals.
http://www.binetusa.org/; 800-585-9368

GLAAD Media Reference Guide – Transgender Issues. An extensive
media reference guide covering transgender issues.
www.glaad.org/reference/transgender

TransgenderZone.com. A transgender medical and social information database.
www.transgenderzone.com/transpanic.htm

Religion for Parents: Videos

Karslake, Daniel, *For the Bible Tells Me So*, First Run Features, 2007.
This documentary on the intersection of religion and homosexuality in the United States focuses on the ways conservative Christians often interpret the Bible in order to deny homosexuals equal
rights.

Logan, Kate, *Kidnapped for Christ, www.kidnappedforchrist.com.* This is a fascinating documentary about conversion therapy.

Vines, Matthew, *https://www.youtube.com/user/vinesmatthew.* These lectures empower LGBT-affirming Christians in nonaffirming churches. Matthew Vines is the founder of the Reformation Project and author of *God and the Gay Christian.*

Support for Accepting Gays & Lesbians Within One's Religion

There is an organization for every religion. This is just a sampling.

Affirmation (Methodist)

Affirmation (Mormon)
www.affirmation.org

Dignity (Catholic)
www.dignityusa.org

Gay Jews (Orthodox)
www.GayJews.org

Political /Current Events

The Advocate
www.advocate.com

BuzzFeed LGBT
www.buzzfeed.com/lgbt

Gay and Lesbian Alliance Against Defamation (GLAAD) (in media)
www.glaad.org

Huffington Post Gay Voices
www.huffingtonpost.com/gayvoices

Human Rights Campaign
www.hrc.org

IGLHRC (International Gay and Lesbian Human Rights
   Commission)

www.outrightinternational.org/National Gay & Lesbian Task Force
   (NGLBTF)
www.ngltf.org

Towle Road
www.towleroad.com

Sexuality Medical Information

Centers for Disease Control and Prevention's LGBT Youth Health
   Center
www.cdc.gov/lgbthealth/youth.htm

SIECUS (Sexuality Information and Education Council of the
   United States)
www.siecus.orgdelete

LGBT Associations

CenterLink: The national association of gay, lesbian, bisexual and
   transgender community centers.
www.lgbtcenters.org

LGBT Support

Association of Gay & Lesbian Psychiatrists
www.aglp.org

GLBT National Helpline: National Hotlinefor information, referral,
   and peer counseling.
www.glbthotline.org/national-hotline.html
   1-888-843-4564

Trevor Hotline: A 24-hour, toll-free, and confidential suicide hotline
   for gay and questioning youth
www.thetrevorproject.org
   1-866-488-7386

Support for Youth

About.com for LGBT Teens
Gayteens.about.com

Empty Closets: Information, peer support, and one-on-one peer
   counseling.
www.emptyclosets.com

Gay Christian
www.gaychristian.net

GLBTnearme.org: A listing of over 15,000 LGBT resources.
www.glbtnearme.org

It Gets Better Project
www.Itgetsbetter.org

Metropolitan Community Church: A gay-friendly church with locations around the world.
www.ufmcc.com

Youth Guardian Services for thirteen- to twenty-five-year-olds
www.youth-guard.org

Bibliography

Bernstein, R.A. *Straight Parents, Gay Children: Inspiring Families to Live Honestly and with Greater Understanding.* New York: Thunder's Mouth Press, 2003.

Dees, Abby. *Queer Questions Straight Talk: 108 Frank & Provocative Questions It's OK to Ask Your Lesbian, Gay, or Bisexual Loved One.* Pittsburgh: St. Lynn's Press, 2010.

DeGeneres, Betty. *Love, Ellen: A Mother/Daughter Journey.* New York: William Morrow, 1999.

Fairchild, Betty, and Nancy Hayward. *Now That You Know: A Parent's Guide to Understanding Their Gay and Lesbian Children.* New York: Harcourt Brace, 1989.

Goldman, Linda. *Coming Out, Coming In: Nurturing the Well-Being and Inclusion of Gay Youth in Mainstream Society.* New York: Routledge, 2008.

Griffin, Carolyn Welch, Marian J. Wirth, and Arthur G. Wirth. *Beyond Acceptance: Parents of Lesbians and Gays Talk About Their Experiences.* New York: St. Martin's Press, 1996.

Isay, Richard A., MD. *Becoming Gay: The Journey of Self-Acceptance.* New York: Vintage, 2009.

Jennings, Kevin, PhD, with Pat Shapiro, MSW. *Always My Child: A Parent's Guide to Understanding Your Gay, Lesbian, Bisexual, Transgendered or Questioning Son or Daughter.* New York: Fireside Press, 2003.

LaSala, Michael C., PhD. *Coming Out, Coming Home.* New York: Columbia University Press, 2010.

Marcus, Eric. *Is It a Choice? Answers to 300 of the Most Frequently Asked Questions About Gay and Lesbian People.* New York: HarperCollins, 1999.

Owens-Reid, Dannielle, and Kristin Russo. *This Is a Book for Parents of Gay Kids.* San Francisco: Chronicle Books, 2014.

Savage, Dan, and Terry Miller, eds. *It Gets Better: Coming Out, Overcoming Bullying, and Creating a Life Worth Living.* New York: Penguin, 2011.

Savin-Williams, Ritch C. *Mom, Dad I'm Gay: How Families Negotiate Coming Out.* Washington, DC: American Psychological Association, 2001.

Savin-Williams, Ritch C. *The New Gay Teenager.* Cambridge: Harvard University Press, 2005.

Schwartz, John. *Oddly Normal: Our Family's Struggle to Help Their Teenage Son Come to Terms with His Sexuality.* New York: Penguin, 2012.

Signorile, Michelangelo. *It's Not Over: Getting Beyond Tolerance, Defeating Homophobia, and Winning True Equality.* Boston: Houghton Mifflin Harcourt, 2015.

Wagner, Paul, and Hjordy Wagner. *Ready or Not . . . THEY'RE GAY: Stories from a Midwest Family.* Austin, Texas: Synergy Books, 2009.

Acknowledgments

From Wesley

I would like to thank all the straight parents and gay/lesbian adults, the latter from teens to forty, who contributed to this book. Whether your interview is contained herein or, due to space constraints, does not appear, your experiences guided me immeasurably in the writing of *When Your Child Is Gay*, as well as in the understanding of the issues inherent in raising gay children. I carry your comments in my head and heart.

I am indebted to my coauthor Jonathan L. Tobkes, MD, who despite a private practice, an affiliation with New York-Presbyterian Weill Cornell Medical Center, a marriage, and two young children in tow, managed to stay ahead of me! I thank Cason Crane, who wrote the wonderful Foreword. I am grateful to Daniel Garza, MD, consulting psychiatrist at Callen-Lorde, for his initial exploration with me of the issues that straight parents and their gay children face.

I am eternally grateful to my editor at Sterling, Kate Zimmermann, for her steadfast diligence, wisdom, and extended hand to a first-time author. My gratitude to Steven Harris of CSG Literary, who saw potential in the proposal I pitched at the American Society of Journalists and Authors' Conference, trusted his gut, and found a suitable publisher in a short time! I thank my-friend-since-the-tenth-grade Lesley Starbuck, actress and life coach, who role-played with me to perfect my pitch for agents. To my publicist Janet Appel, I thank you for your seasoned advice for markets to get the message out there! I am grateful to my mentor Phyllis Schneider, whose experience in the magazine field helped me to make the transition from advertising copywriter to journalism.

Of course, a book starts with a proposal. I'd like to thank those who helped me fashion one: Jennifer Lawler, Diane O'Connell, Beverly West, Dawn Hardy, and David Kohn. I would still be writing *Resources for Straight Families and LGBT Adults* were it not for Susan Berner and Mirje Heide.

To all my English teachers at Rosemary Hall (now Choate Rosemary Hall) who made us write, write, write, and diagram sentences; I am beholden to you. You actually taught us grammar! To my sister Dr. Dancy Kittrell who helped me organize my thoughts for this book. To my other sister Betsy Cullen who brainstormed more concepts with me than a creative agency team at an advertising agency!

I'm eternally grateful that my husband had the foresight to build a house with "a room of my own" for writing. Since we met on January 29, 1972, he somehow knows when to leave me alone to compose and when to give me a hug!

But most of all, I thank our son. He has shown us that it's

possible to alter your expectations when love is involved. It has been an ongoing journey, and I'm the better for it. I have been privileged to glimpse into a world that I would not ordinarily have seen had it not been for you. Thank you for the honor!

From Jonathan

First and foremost, I would like to thank my loving husband, Tad Tobkes, who not only initially connected me with coauthor Wesley Davidson, but who also encouraged and supported me through every single step of this project. Tad's boundless positivity, altruism, and passion for life inspire me on a daily basis. I couldn't feel more proud or fortunate to be spending my life, and to be creating a family, with him.

I am forever indebted to coauthor, Wesley Davidson, who conceptualized and outlined this book long before my involvement, and who carefully guided me through the process of my first manuscript. I truly admire her indefatigable work ethic and tenacity.

I would like to give a special thank you to my former elementary school teacher, Michael Yosha, who believed in me long before I believed in myself. He instilled in me the crucial lifelong lesson of never giving up, taught me to love myself as I am, and showed me that there are no limits to what I can accomplish.

I am deeply grateful to Linda Knier, my unconditionally supportive and ever helpful mother-in-law and fellow grammarian, who dropped everything in the middle of her busy weeks to offer feedback and commentary on my chapter form and content.

My close friend and colleague, Atara Stahl, urged me to write this book when I expressed concern that there weren't enough hours in the day. For the last decade, she has been my rock and confidante. Amazingly, there isn't a problem she cannot solve.

Daniel Yadegar gives new meaning to the term loyal. His incisive feedback was incredibly helpful and is always appreciated.

Everyone should be so lucky as to have Scott Goldsmith's compassionate and brilliant mentorship to usher them through the coming-out process, and then his continuing support and friendship to guide them through all of the amazing life events that follow.

Finally, there would be no book without my patients. They are an infinite source of inspiration and motivation to me, and I am forever grateful to them for sharing themselves and their lives with me. I feel incredibly blessed to be a psychiatrist, and I so deeply cherish the supreme privilege of working with each and every one of my patients.

About the Authors

WESLEY DAVIDSON graduated from Rosemary Hall, a secondary school, then in Greenwich, Connecticut, now merged with The Choate School in Wallingford, Connecticut. In the eighth grade, she won the English Prize, for which she received a watercolor copy of Santiago, the old man, catching the marlin from Hemingway's *Old Man and the Sea*. The original went to Ernest Hemingway. It hangs in her home office in Vero Beach.

A graduate of Finch College in New York City with a major in Art History, Wesley, during college, was Co-chairman of Finch's Art Museum where she was photographed for *Newsweek* magazine. After college, she worked in art galleries, but decided after a few years to turn her efforts towards writing.

She attended New York University, the New School, and School of Visual Arts to learn the craft of copywriting and magazine writing. She worked in advertising and public relations for various firms in New York City and Westchester County, where she and her husband John lived for twenty-five years as they raised two children, James, thirty-two, who is gay, and Ann, now, twenty-seven. Wesley wrote health and parenting articles for parenting and national publications, including *Good Housekeeping*, *American Baby*, and *Adoptive Families*.

She now lives in Vero Beach, Florida, with her husband, John.

JONATHAN L. TOBKES, MD, is a practicing psychiatrist in New York City, whose patients include many gay and lesbian people as well as the straight parents of lesbians and gays. He was born and raised in Baldwin, New York (graduating as valedictorian from Baldwin Senior High School), followed by Yale University (from which he graduated cum laude with a distinction in his major) and NYU School of Medicine (where he was a member of AOA Honor Society). He completed his residency in adult psychiatry at Payne Whitney Clinic at Weill Cornell Medical Center and then a child/adolescent psychiatry fellowship at NYU Child Study Center. He currently teaches and supervises psychiatry residents at The New York-Presbyterian/Weill Cornell Medical Center in Manhattan. He lives in New York City with his husband, Taylor, and their two children, Samson and Hannah.

Index